My Life with Phil

The dramatic forgotten story behind the world's first successful heart transplant

By Eileen Blaiberg
as told to
Graham Fysh

Published by Lifetime Creations, Silverdale, Washington, USA

ISBN: 979-8-9854836-7-3

Author's Note

When Dr. Philip Blaiberg became the world's first successful heart transplant recipient in 1968 I was selected to cover the ups and downs of his newfound life for *The Cape Argus*, where I worked. I spent many days with Phil and his wife Eileen. My reports, including those written for the series *Dr. Blaiberg Day By Day,* appeared in newspapers around the world.

When Phil died Eileen asked me to write her story. We called her story *My Life with Phil*. It was to be published by a major U.S. publisher. With the help of my wife Marcia I put it together in six weeks. Delays by lawyers and others in sending the book to the publisher led to their rejecting it as, they said, world interest in the topic would have waned by the time it came out in print. I did succeed, however, in publishing it in Italian under the title *Ho vissuto con un risuscitato*.

I kept the original manuscript of *My Life with Phil* for 56 years over many moves across two continents.

Now here it is, with a few additions that I have added from other material that I kept—all in Eileen's words. Preserved for you to read.

The Blaiberg transplant performed by Dr. Barnard was indeed pioneering. Today about 5,000 successful heart transplants are performed around the world each year. The transplant, however, exacted a toll on Eileen that only a few people have ever had to endure. More than 56 years later, therefore, the story remains as dramatic and gripping as it was then.

I trust you will enjoy it.

— Graham Fysh

1

Cape Town, South Africa June 19, 1955: It was our son Harris's 17th birthday. We went out for dinner. Phil had a colossal meal.

We returned home about one o'clock in the morning. Phil got into bed and read for about an hour.

Then it happened. The attack came quietly, unheralded, like a vulture swooping down on its unsuspecting prey. One minute Phil lay next to me, reading his newspaper. The next minute great drops of perspiration appeared on his brow.

He turned to me, clearly in agony, but fully in control.

"Eileen, I am having a heart attack. Call the doctor. Tell him to come immediately because I am very ill."

I ran to the telephone.

The wait was agonising, more physically painful for Phil, but equally tense for us both. He grit his teeth, unable to hide the pain. His body was wet from perspiration now.

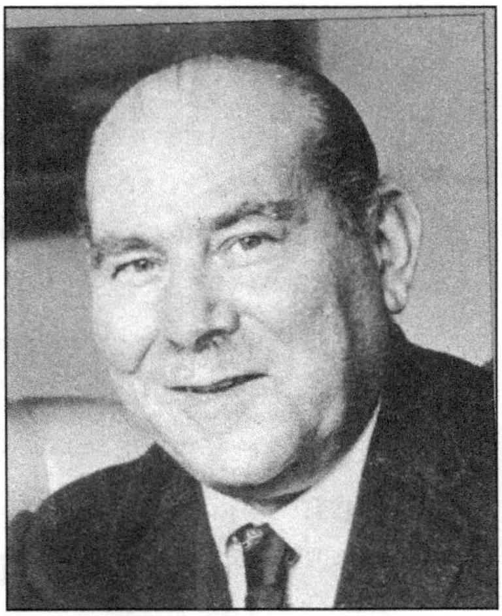
Dr. Philip Blaiberg

"I wish he would come. If he does not come soon, it will be all over," he said.

"Nonsense," I replied, knowing nevertheless that all the symptoms were there. He was throwing up. An excruciating pain spread across his chest and into his left arm.

When Dr. Wilfred Kohn, our family doctor, came 10 minutes later Phil was in intense pain, but he still had not panicked in any way.

"Wilfred," he said. "This is it, old boy. I've got a beautiful coronary. Give me the strongest injection you can to take away the pain."

Relaxed relief settled on him as the injection took effect.

The doctor called me aside and said the attack was a severe posterior coronary and I should steel myself for the worst, which might happen at any time.

The pain was suppressed, but he was still in the clasp of that swooping vulture that was to make more attacks on him and was to weaken him still further in the future.

Above all, I suffered a psychological blow along with Phil. Until then, I had taken health for granted. You know how it is, you string along in a carefree way, happy to be alive and not really touched by the troubles of others. It will never happen to you, you say. Then the halcyon days are gone, snatched from you forever. Those birthdays you were not counting any longer rush in to give account of themselves.

The fresh vigour of youth melts in the harsh glare of the afternoon sun. Suddenly evening is before you, the night prepared to spring from the shadows. The good times are a memory of the morning, the lengthening shade the reality of the present.

Those 10 minutes of agony changed the whole pivot of our lives. Our hopes and fears of yesterday were not our hopes and fears of today. More heart attacks were to come in the years ahead and Phil was to come even closer to death.

Little did we know then, however, that a near-miraculous event lay on the horizon. That event was to change our lives in a dramatic way that was impossible to foresee or even imagine.

But let me start at the beginning. That will set the stage for all that Phil and I went through before we faced the unbelievable.

2

We were heading for the golf course that night in the early 1930s. The darkness was closing in on us as we drove along the unlit, lonely country road.

It had been their idea—the young man driving the car and his fellow golfing buddy. Both were getting ready to leave their homes in the small South African country town of Oudtshoorn. Both were golf addicts, and they wanted to say farewell to the golf course. I decided to humour them and join them on the ride.

The three friends, who had just emerged from adolescence into their twenties, laughed as they drove toward the golf course. What a silly idea, they said, to say goodbye to a golf course.

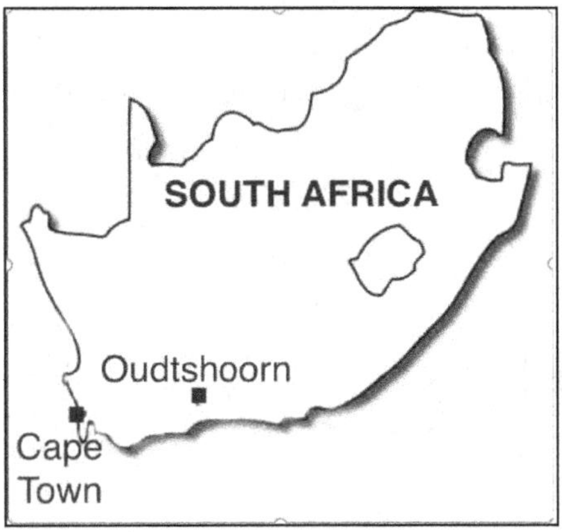

Who does that? They did.

Suddenly a lonely figure at the side of the road appeared in the car's headlights and waved to them to stop. He appeared to me to be a tramp. I was nervous. "Don't stop," I said. "He looks as though he might be dangerous."

"I don't think so," replied the driver. "He looks quite respectable to me." His friend agreed.

The driver braked. The "tramp" climbed into the car.

"Hullo," he said. "My name is Philip Blaiberg."

I was taken aback. So here was Philip Blaiberg in the flesh, sitting right next to me in the back of the car. Not only was he no tramp, but he also was a rugby player whose name was a household word in Oudtshoorn. In addition he came with rugged good looks.

I had admired him in the past. Now he was right next to me. And, as far as he was concerned, I might as well not exist.

"My mother is alone in the car," Phil quickly explained to the men in the front of the car. "One of the tyres is flat and I don't have the tools to repair it. I left her there and started walking to find help.

"I had already walked quite a long way in this direction when you drove past. I'm so pleased you stopped for me. I'm getting worried about my mother sitting alone in the car in the dark."

Along the way my thoughts turned back to a time eight years before. I had seen Phil then, although his actions in the car showed that he clearly did not remember me. The truth was, however, that I had taken more than a passing interest in the broad, blonde-haired rugby star. He was not simply one of the crowd in the town of Oudtshoorn. He was, I recalled, strikingly different, a cut above the rest, endowed with good looks, talent and intelligence.

He had turned my head that day as he walked down the street. I had stopped and stared at him. But I immediately dismissed any thoughts of getting to know him better. After all I was only 12 and he was 16. At that age the gap between us was almost as wide as a generation. Most of the boys I mixed with were no older than 14. He was out of the age of eligibility and simply unattainable.

In any event Phil seemed more interested in sport than in girls.

I thought back, too, to the time when one evening Phil's school athletic team staged a display of physical culture. He took my breath away as he performed gymnastic feats and pulled himself along on the parallel bars. He was the star of the whole performance for me.

Yet he could be no more than an idolised hero.

Unattainable.

One day Phil actually approached me in the street. I wondered what he was going to say. It came as quite an anti-climax when he said, "My younger brother is crazy about you."

Disappointed, I retorted, "Go and tell your younger brother to jump in the lake."

"What about me?" he asked.

"Well, that's different. We won't discuss that now."

Phil failed to detect any hint in my answer. He walked off.

Unattainable.

Tonight sitting alongside me in the car Phil had forgotten that incident, I concluded. Did he not even realise I was in the car? Could he not even have greeted me?

Unattainable.

Before too long the car's headlights picked up Phil's car at the side of the road. His mother was waiting patiently. The young men got out of the car. They found the necessary tools in Phil's car. Soon they were working on changing the wheel.

"Well, what a surprise," said a somewhat embarrassed Phil. "Fancy that. The tools were in the car all the time. You see, I have been living in England for four years and I did not own a car over there. I had no idea that cars are now equipped with these tools."

Huh. A poor excuse, I thought. What a blithering idiot. He let his mother Gertrude sit in the dark in the car all that time without even looking inside the vehicle for the tools to change the wheel. He probably did not know how to change the wheel anyway.

The friends continued on their way to the golf course, leaving Phil to drive his mother home.

As my friends bade farewell to their beloved golf course, my thoughts flooded back again to those days shortly after I had just celebrated my thirteenth birthday. In Oudtshoorn in those days a group of teenage boys established what they called a "club." A rule of the club was anyone who did not greet them in the way they deemed to be proper would be boycotted.

I remembered that I had been boycotted for two weeks because I failed to observe the rule.

But Phil did not belong to the club. He regarded it as foolish and childish. He was mature beyond his years. A thinker and a philosopher, at the age of 17 he was more adult than his contemporaries.

Much of Phil's approach to life, even at that early age, came from his parents. His father loved education and learning. Indeed, he spent so much time reading and discussing philosophy that he seldom was concerned about the hum-drum business of making a living. He left that to Phil's mother who was a business-like, practical woman.

Eventually Phil's mother took over the bread-winning side of the family completely, and she made a good job of it. So much so that she was a wealthy woman when she died.

Phil admired his father, Jacob, who inspired him to study and seek out the deeper things in life. But he also admired his mother for her practical hard work. He inherited the best attributes of both his parents—a philosopher who also would knuckle down and perform the work required of him.

Many a 16- or 17-year-old in Oudtshoorn in those days was something of an introvert and an egotist. Teens were concerned above all else about their own appearances, about how others viewed them, and about their own interests. Typical teenagers also were rebels, disinterested in the views or achievements of their elders.

Phil was not your typical 17-year-old, however. He was an extrovert, absorbed in the interests of others. Parties were a waste of time for him. He was more serious-minded than the average youth of that age.

He was always probing, finding out, inquiring and learning. He never took anything for granted.

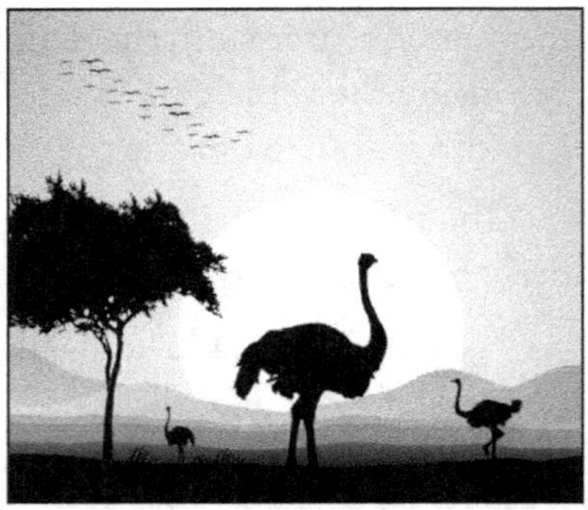

He found a lot to occupy his inquiring mind in the Oudtshoorn of those days. The hub of an area that was home to many ostrich farms, it was the centre of a thriving global trade in ostrich feathers. So much so that it was called "The Little Paris." During the ostrich feather boom a woman who failed to wear ostrich feathers simply was not counted among the better dressed people in society. Money from around the world flowed into the area around Oudtshoorn as did many people looking for prosperity in the ostrich feather trade.

When Phil was in his later teens, the boom was in its dying days, but many immigrants decided to make Oudtshoorn their home even when the boom was over.

Unlike his peers, Phil mixed a lot with adults, listening eagerly to the stories of their lives, eager to know how they came to be in Oudtshoorn. Wanting to know what motivated people, he would ask immigrants why they had chosen to live there, delving at length into the reasons they had made the decision to leave their ancestral homes. He learned stories of Jewish people who had come from Russia, Poland or Germany, accumulating a fund of anecdotes.

He came from a home where people were valued for their own value, not how much money they were worth.

Rugby occupied a lot of his time. He became one of the youngest players to represent South-Western Districts, the region into which Oudtshoorn fell.

Phil's character appealed to me because, in some ways, it was the opposite of mine. I came from a home where snobbery was a way of life. My father, Israel Harris Abel, had been wealthy. So much so he was able to afford the first automobile in the Cape Province. I rode alongside him with pride down the road in the South African town of Paarl, where I grew up.

Then came the financial crash. Facing widespread losses, Israel bought a hotel to keep the family going.

When I was seven, the family moved to East London on the South African east coast where the family lived in one of the hotels my father had bought. Five years later we moved to Oudtshoorn, where again we lived in a hotel that my father owned.

Even into my twenties, I never lived in a home as most people know it. Living full-time in a hotel placed me in something of a spotlight. Young men were often around. I simply could not afford to be badly dressed or untidy.

Just as I entered my teen years, Phil became even more unattainable—at least to me. At the age of 17, after matriculating from an Oudtshoorn school, he left to study at Witwatersrand University in Johannesburg. where he completed his first year of medicine. To qualify as a dentist in those days, however, he needed to go abroad.

He might have been out of sight in Johannesburg, but for me he was not out of mind. The local newspaper regularly carried reports on his progress. After all, he was the epitome of the "local boy made good." He soon was on the first under-19 rugby team at Witwatersrand University in the Johannesburg area.

After a short visit to Oudtshoorn at the end of his first year, he left for Britain to complete his studies in dentistry. He was to spend four years there before qualifying.

Even when he was in England his rugby prowess was eagerly followed by the Oudtshoorn newspaper. He became captain of the Royal Dental Hospital rugby team where he became one of the first South Africans to captain an overseas rugby team.

Phil showed prowess in England in another respect, too. The good-looking rugby star was not shy when it came to the fairer sex.

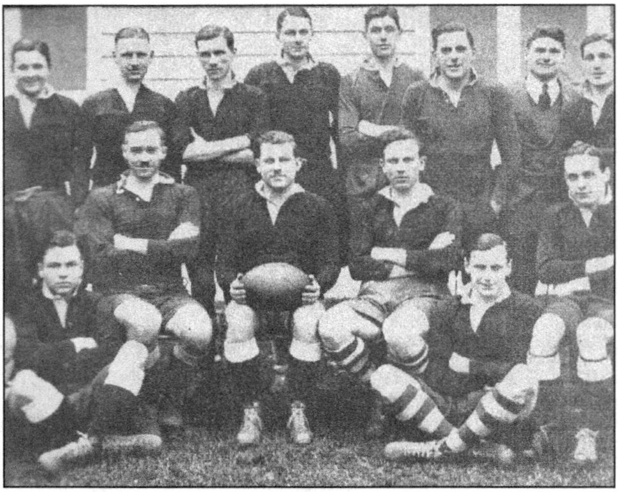

Phil (with ball), as rugby team captain

He developed quite a reputation while he was in London. Even his landlady complained about the girls he would bring into the boarding house.

When he returned to Oudtshoorn the news soon spread: Philip Blaiberg is back in town. His mother, who was successfully running a local store, was like a child with a new toy when Phil returned. She had been unable to visit him in England. The fares were too expensive and the main way to get there was by ship. Not only that, but the trip itself would take a long time; saving for the fare took even longer.

He returned to an enthusiastic welcome home. Philip Blaiberg—aged 23 and a strapping young man with a promising future—was back. A hero who had returned to his home town. It was one of the social events of the year in Oudtshoorn.I watched these events at a distance.

Phil's mother had bought up the equipment of a dentist who had become bankrupt in a small village named Robertson, 170 miles (270 km) west of Oudtshoorn. She had heard about the sale from a dental company and, always one with an eye for a bargain, thought this would be ideal for her son, eager to start his own dental practice.

Phil took up her offer and moved to Robertson, but refused further help from his mother. He had a proud independent spirit. He would take it from there, even though he knew it would be a struggle. After all, dentists earned little in the 1930s and the Robertson population from which he could draw clients was small.

Phil struggled to adapt himself to the quiet pace of the small village.

He spent his time off in the hotel where he stayed, playing cards and drinking with friends. He made regular visits to Oudtshoorn where, although its size was far from that of a city, offered a faster pace of life.

In contrast with London, Robertson was a true backwater.

I had followed his progress, but at a distance. I had not seen Phil since he left for London almost five years before.

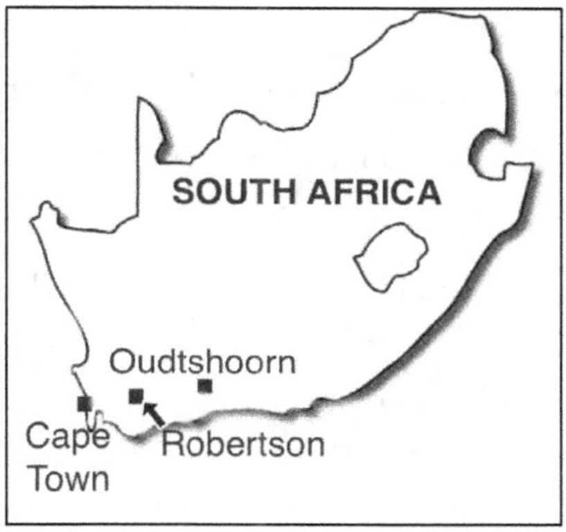

The turning point came one evening when Phil returned on a visit to Oudtshoorn a few weeks after his move to Robertson. He attended the movies with a friend.

I happened to be in the cinema that evening. My heart leaped when I caught sight of the handsome young man sitting on the opposite side of the aisle from me. I noticed he was eyeing me.

"Who is that?" I asked my friend.

"Don't you know?" my friend replied. "That is Philip Blaiberg."

Of course it was. Was he now attainable?

"Better lay off," my friend continued. I hear he has a girl friend."

Nevertheless, during the intermission, Phil walked up to me.

"Have we met before?" he asked.

"Yes. I'm Eileen Abel."

Phil replied that he was a little disappointed to hear we were already acquainted.

"I thought you were a nice young thing I could take out to have a good time with," he continued, with a twinkle in his eye. "Now that I realise we already know one another, it makes it a bit awkward."

The conversation ended there; the movie was about to start.

Still unattainable.

Phil returned to Oudtshoorn for the Yom Kippur (Day of Atonement) services. Wearing a long red dress and sitting in a seat in the upper row of the synagogue, I felt someone was looking at me from the men's section downstairs. I resisted the temptation to look down, but eventually had to give in. My heart skipped a beat when I saw it was Phil looking up at me.

"You are not going to get away from me this time," I thought as the service droned on. The woman sitting alongside me—who clearly had watched the eyeing across the levels—said as I got out of my seat, "Let me know when the engagement is announced."

We met as we made our way out of the synagogue.

"May I have the pleasure of walking you home?" Phil asked.

Attainable? Maybe.

God must have sanctioned that encounter in the synagogue, I believed. While there I had prayed about nothing else. There could be no turning back.

Courting was not easy for Phil and me. After all, he lived in another town almost a three-hour drive away where he had to continue his work as a dentist. It was out of the question for me to leave Oudtshoorn and move to Robertson.

We resorted to occasional visits, letters and long-distance telephone calls, which were expensive in those days. Our long-distance courtship continued for two-and-a-half years. During that time many friends asked, "When are you two going to become engaged?" But Phil and I both knew there was little purpose in becoming engaged until Phil had built up his practice and was earning a comfortable income on which we both could live. We ignored the hints. We continued telephoning and writing.

Phil faced an uphill battle in Robertson building up a sizable practice. He faced competition from two dentists who were established in the town. Indeed, the size of the town did not merit more than two dentists anyway. Not only that, but his predecessor had become bankrupt.

Work grew gradually, however. Phil worked hard and conscientiously. Over time, the results started showing. As the practice started to flourish we looked forward to a happy life together. The wedding day, it seemed, was not far off.

Then the first big tragedy of my life struck.

3

My father Israel was an ill man. He had suffered many years from diabetes, for which there was no treatment in those days. Insulin was discovered only toward the end of his life. He then received many injections of insulin, but it did not seem to help that much.

So much so that I could never remember my father being a well man. It was sometimes a struggle for him just to stand. It was sad for me to see him suffer in that way.

Phil reminded me of my father. At that time, however, I had no idea just how similar the two men would be. History repeated itself. Our daughter, Jill, also had her share of having a father who suffered for a considerable length of time.

Not only in being ill, but also in other ways, Israel and Phil were remarkably alike.

My father, too, was a distinctive man, one who stood out from the rest. He was straight-forward, always making clear exactly where you stood with him. Both were philosophers who liked to sit for hours and discuss the deeper mysteries of life.

Their standards were based on the kind of person you were, no matter your background. Both refused to discriminate against people, but at the same time were not excessive fraternisers either.

Perhaps that was why Phil and I became the best of friends. My father was to say that he would prefer Phil to almost any other young man in Oudtshoorn to be his son-in-law.

When he was so ill, my father wanted to return to his native Czechoslovakia. He believed that the well-known Carlsbad Baths in that country would do him a lot of good. Stays for several weeks with regular visits to the thermal hot springs and spas were said to heal visitors and improve their health.

Famous European composers and aristocrats—including Johann Wolfgang Goethe, Frederick Chopin, and Peter the Great—helped make the town of Karlovy Vary, known in English as Carlsbad Baths, highly popular.

Believing he needed help in making the visit, my father asked me to accompany him.

The decision was a difficult one for me. Two fares would be straining the family's finances. And, more importantly, I would be away from Phil.

Above all I was madly in love with Phil yet able to telephone him in Robertson only now and then and to write to him occasionally. Those communications were poor substitutes for being with him, but the situation would be considerably worse from as far away as Czechoslovakia.

I was part of a large family—I had five sisters and two brothers—yet, although 22, I was the only one who could make the trip. My older sisters were married and my brother was managing the hotel on which the family depended for income.

I thought carefully. Finally I decided to stay in South Africa.

It was a decision I regretted for the rest of my life.

When I thought in later years that my father went alone to Carlsbad without any of his seven children with him, I often wanted to cry. The reason: My father died at Carlsbad. All alone.

"I should have gone with him," I tearfully said in later years. "After all, I was to have many years to be close to Phil. But going to Carlsbad would be the last chance I would have had to be close to my father."

4

Two-and-a-half months after my father died I was still upset about his death and my failure to join him in Czechoslovakia. Phil sensed this was the right time to take my mind off the tragedy and focus on happier times.

From that night in the synagogue our romance blossomed. I lived from one long weekend to the next. We wrote love letters and telephoned each other regularly.

But between his visits I was terribly lonely. In those days the car journey between Robertson and Oudtshoorn was long and dreary, with shocking roads, and two steep mountain passes.

We both felt so far from each other.

The highlight of our courtship of two years, which to a young girl seemed much longer, was our first holiday together at a pleasant little seaside resort, Mossel Bay, about 60 miles from Oudtshoorn.

In those days young people were more aware of the conventions than they are now. We booked at different hotels so that it would appear we met by chance instead of by arrangement.

We had never been together before for as long as 10 days; and well do I remember our swims in the sea, the hikes, picnics, and dancing at hotels by night to the popular tune of the time, "Smoke Gets In Your Eyes". We danced to it, looking into each other's eyes. Perhaps that is why we were voted, by holiday-makers, the most romantic couple of the season. They could see we were so much in love. Whenever I hear that tune today, it reminds me still of those happy, halcyon days at Mossel Bay.

Although we both accepted that we would eventually marry, we never discussed a definite wedding date. Phil was building up a practice at Robertson and not earning sufficient money to support a wife. Sometimes my parents wondered whether our courtship would ever end in marriage.

I reassured them. "Don't worry. We must have patience. One of these days Phil will be on his feet, and he'll be able to afford to marry."

Nevertheless, as the months and years passed I began to wonder, as my parents did, whether Phil would ever give me an engagement ring and announce our impending marriage.

Not long after my father died in August 1935 Phil came to Oudtshoorn to sympathize with our family. He told me he had a big surprise for me. Womanlike, I demanded to know what it was. He wouldn't tell me. All in good time, he said.

That night he drove me to a quiet spot outside the town. It was full moon and as bright as day. Putting his hand in his pocket he drew out a number of diamond rings that flashed in the moonlight.

"Take your choice." he grinned. I chose a beautiful solitaire and put it on.

"It's lovely, Phil." I cried, "It's the most marvellous gift I've ever had. Oh, you've made me so happy!"

We kissed and lay in each other's arms talking of the future, the happiness we would know together, and of all the wonderful things lovers speak of at such precious and unforgettable moments in their lives.

We got home in the early hours of the morning. I woke up my mother, sisters, and brother to tell them the wonderful news. There was no need to announce the engagement. Next day the entire community of Oudtshoorn knew of it and turned up to congratulate us. Telegrams began to stream in.

"Mazeltov," one read. "So you're going to marry the blithering idiot after all."

'The idiot' and I had the distinction of seeing our wedding photograph in the intaglio (gravure) section of The Cape Times.

We were described as among "The Couples of the Year".

Photographs of country weddings rarely appeared in the city newspapers in South Africa in those days. What a send-off that was on our honeymoon.

We were married in the Oudtshoorn Synagogue on April 5, 1936.

Phil and I did not plan any festivities, but our friends wanted to make sure we celebrated the occasion.

They arrived at the hotel where I lived and were ready to party. I said the time was not yet ready for parties. My father's death still hung heavily over me.

"Please talk quietly," I said. "Don't sing and dance. I want to respect my father's memory and I feel a deep sense of loss and regret."

Nevertheless, our friends only went so far as to keep the merriment subdued.

Even at the wedding, I requested that there be no dancing.

"My father died eight months ago and I still do not want too much merry-making," I said. "I feel it is out of place."

At the wedding Phil's father, Jacob Blaiberg, delivered a speech that I was to remember for the rest of my life. He said that, according to the Talmud, the Jewish book of learning, one should never be jealous of one's son. Yet he admitted he was jealous of his son that day.

"I am a little envious that my son is taking a more clever step than I did," he said. "He is 26. I became married when I was much older—in my forties. That means he can become a father at a much younger age. I have so many regrets that I am so much older than my eldest son."

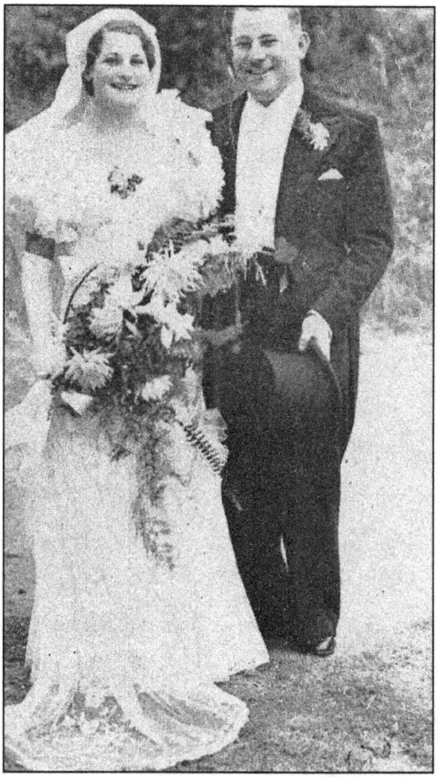

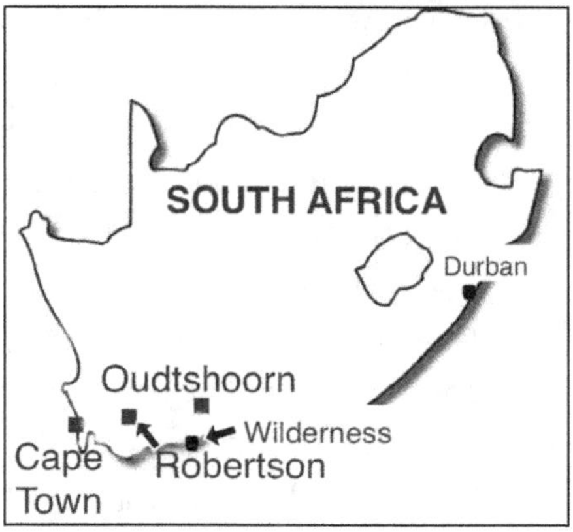

Jacob was approaching 70 at the time of the wedding and was also a lot older than his wife.

We spent our honeymoon at the Wilderness, a coastal town in the south-eastern area of South Africa, surrounded by the bounties of nature. A lack of money led to the honeymoon being short. Although Phil's mother, Gertrude Leah Portnoi, had made a success of her business and

Phil's parents were considered moneyed people, Phil was insistent that whatever he was going to achieve he was going to achieve himself.

In those days it was difficult to make ends meet financially.

The situation is illustrated in a humorous story.

My sister and her husband suggested that, because they had such a short honeymoon, they should accompany us a little later on a trip up the coast to Durban.

"Eileen," Phil replied. "The only trip you will have being married to a dentist is in a canoe up the Breede River at Robertson."

During our married life we developed adages that helped to keep us happily married and prevented arguments and bitterness.

Phil taught me one of those on the first night of our honeymoon.

"Never go to sleep on your quarrels," he said. "An old lady told me this is one of the secrets to a happy marriage and we are going to stick to that."

And so we did. For all 33 years of our married lives.

Phil wore the pants in our home in no uncertain way. He was the boss and he showed it.

When he made up his mind about a matter it became past discussion. I, however, was happy to let him lead. If I disagreed with anything that Phil said I knew I would lose anyway. So rather than prolong the quarrel, I gave in fairly easily and would fit in with what he said.

Indeed, Phil was obstinate at times. Once he made up his mind there was no way he would change it. When he was older, however, he mellowed and was not quite as obstinate as at the start of our life together.

He learned there could be times when black was not always black nor white always white. The truth lay somewhere in between in a pale shade of gray.

We lived in a hotel in Robertson and I did not work. My whole world, therefore, centered around our marriage. I would get hurt easily when Phil said something that I did not like. Phil would not give in to me, however. No hugging, kissing, or "I'll take you out for dinner tonight." Phil was as solid as concrete in the face of my tears.

He did not believe one should pamper or spoil a person. I learned to become independent. I had to stand on my own two feet.

We did have a particularly bitter quarrel one night, however. A number of travelers regularly stayed at the hotel and ate dinner there. Inevitably, some of them had known Phil before he and I were married. Phil often invited them to sit at our table.

One night Phil and his guests paid no attention to me at all. Not only did Phil ignore me, but he told the guests how much he envied them being bachelors. I felt embarrassed and humiliated.

The final insult came when I left the table in an angry mood. Phil failed to follow me upstairs to our room as I thought he would.

Alone in the room I became more and more outraged. When Phil finally retired to the room, I was packing my suitcase—or at least pretending to do so.

"I am going back to my mother," I shouted, tears streaming down my face.

Phil quietly undressed and climbed into bed.

"Don't you care if I go back to my mother?"

"What are you going to do for money for the train? I certainly am not going to give you any."

That broke the tension. I laughed. I realised I was being ridiculous. We made up and kept to our adage: "Never go to sleep on your quarrels."

Another adage we shared was to share a double bed. We were horrified to hear of couples who slept in single beds. Apart from sex, we believed you cannot help but have love, comradeship and closeness in your lives if you are close together when you sleep.

"It is so easy," I later recalled, "to stretch out your hand and show your husband or wife that you care. Single beds cause troubles to grow and increase the tension because a simple hug or kiss is not that easy when you are in single beds."

That is a reason I believed we were a particularly happily married couple. As the years passed our love for one another deepened.

We noticed, for example, that when other couples reached their forties or fifties they seldom said, "I love you" to one another—at least in front of other people. Perhaps, I thought, they said that to each other when they were alone. But Phil and I often said that even in front of others.

An additional secret of our happy marriage was what I called "reciprocity." We learned from one another, adjusting our way of life to fit in with that of the other—forgiving, forgetting, compensating. We were constantly giving and taking from one another.

At first, Phil had no time for romance or any form of sentimentality. He never brought me flowers now and then, for example. But he learned over the years that a woman expected sentimentality in her life and that it should be an important part of one's marriage.

So it was that I waited in suspense for weeks in advance before I celebrated my 23rd birthday a month after we were married. What, I thought, was he going to give me for my birthday? Surely it would be something special. After all, he would be eager to impress me. It was to be the most exciting day since we had become married.

The big day dawned and the shock came. He gave me nothing. No flowers, no present. It was just the same as any other day—except he did wish me a happy birthday.

Phil returned home from work to find me crying bitterly. He was puzzled.

"What is the matter? Why are you crying?"

"Oh, Phil. It's my birthday. You didn't buy me anything."

"But you know you can go and buy yourself anything on my account at any time you like."

"You don't understand. You don't understand what a woman feels like on her birthday. I expect a present."

Phil tried to explain that, as far as he was concerned, you never communicated through flowers. If you loved your wife, there was no need to do anything special to show her that. She would sense it from every action every day. You would care for her, love her all the time. Even a birthday present was unnecessary.

Phil explained that his action was not through a lack of love. To him, simply saying "many happy returns" was sufficient.

He was used to being straight with people. He told them exactly how he felt. Never did he try to hold out flowers with one hand and get ready to throw a bomb at you with the other hand.

His approach was simply saying "happy birthday" and meaning it, he added. He did not have to prove it by sending flowers, a card and a big fat birthday present.

I accepted that what he said was, to a large extent, true. I saw that flowers and birthday presents were in themselves unimportant. More important things counted in life.

I failed to accept it entirely, however. I persuaded Phil to accept that flowers now and then were important as a gesture—an expression of how you felt in a different way.

We achieved a compromise. The secret lay in reciprocity—give and take.

More than that. After that Phil never failed to give me a present for my birthday, even though it usually was modest. I responded by keeping my birthday gifts to Phil modest.

After all, a big present was not a substitute for love and care.

Another key to marital happiness, we believed, was to have a joint banking account. We never had separate accounts at any stage of our married life.

This approach had nothing to do with money itself, I explained later. It had a lot to do with mutual trust. He never questioned what I bought on the account or why I bought it. I, in turn, never wasted money.

Another illustration of how we learned to live happily by agreeing to differ was when I tried to teach him how to play Bridge.

I had learned to play Bridge when I was 12. A postmaster who lived at our hotel had taught me and both my sisters how to play the game so he would have people to play with him. Soon we became experts.

After a number of unsuccessful attempts to teach Phil, I decided that if we wanted to stay happily married, I would have to stop teaching him how to play the game.

The problem was that he failed to show interest in the rules of the game and would not concentrate.

While I was explaining the intricacies of Bridge, Phil would say, "I must tell you what happened at rugby practice today," or "Have you read this book?"

The problem was that he believed he could spend his time more profitably reading. He was like a sponge, soaking up information.

To him Bridge was a waste of time.

"It provides no opportunity for relaxing," he said. "And you gain no knowledge from it."

I was quick to disagree.

"You exercise your brain while you are playing," I countered.

His approach angered me. Eventually, however, we came to respect each other's views.

I stopped playing Bridge for three years but later I spent time once a week playing Bridge with friends.

Those early years living in a quiet village off the beaten track proved a great start to our married life.

We were forced to be together for most of the time. We needed to get to know each other. If we could not get on with each other, life would become intolerable.

Certainly we had friends but there was no entertainment to distract us. You had to depend to a great extent on yourselves to provide your own entertainment.

You need to do a lot of adjusting when you marry. We had the time and the opportunity to do that adjusting in Robertson.

The scars of my father's death were healing when the dark shadow of a fanatical ruler was being cast over the world. It reached into the tree-lined avenues of Robertson, too, intruding into our lives.

These intrusions would become all too regular, necessitating a gathering of the threads to try to achieve what we had tasted—a paradise in our own Garden of Eden.

Tasting it and realizing how good it was made it seem too good to be true. Perhaps it *was* too good to be true.

5

Later, I realised that the following years were a training ground for the days when we were to lead lives in the spotlight, when we joined the ranks of the most well-known families in the world at that time.

Most of our friends in Robertson were non-Jewish. We had learned to judge people on the basis of their inherent characteristics no matter their standing in the community. Phil was determined not to pigeon-hole people because of their money or lack of it, because of their religion, their birthplace or for any other reason. People were people who should all be judged on an equal basis without any bias.

At times, however, we were disillusioned when small displays of anti-semitism cropped up in the small, happy community. The displays did not come from our friends. The fact that we kept almost all the non-Jewish friends we made in Robertson for the rest of our lives served as ample testimony.

Nevertheless, we felt an invisible barrier was building around us. Nazism was growing into a powerful force. Its ideas were being propagated around the world. It forced many to ponder our differences in ethnic backgrounds whereas before we had not even thought about them.

Insidiously Nazi propaganda made us become aware of being Jewish more than we had ever felt before, And it made those who were not Jewish more aware, too, that we were Jewish.

Phil and I continued to go to parties and dances in groups, happily enjoying life together. As 1939 approached, however, we felt a coolness invading that happiness.

Phil noticed a changing attitude in his dental practice, too. He could not pinpoint it definitely. Nothing was blatant, biting or bitter. Both he and I perceived the differences in small ways. Often, however, those little things hurt more than the more obvious bigger ones.

We heard of parties to which we had not been invited. The parties were held by people who had invited us before. We sensed why we had not been invited this time.

The more sensitive we became the more irritating the pinpricks became.

Finally Phil and I decided that the time had come to move. We felt we would not feel the pinpricks as much in a bigger city. The interpersonal relationships would be less tense there. We believed the insinuations would be less noticeable.

In short, the less friendly, less parochial atmosphere of a big city would be our ally.

We chose to move to Cape Town.

The move meant starting from scratch. The three years in Robertson were not entirely wasted, however, as Phil obtained a reasonable price for his dental practice.

The move did mean, however, that Phil would have to build a new practice. We would need to find new friends and learn to live a new kind of life.

Not only that. We would start the new life with an additional member of the family. Before we left for Cape Town our son, Harris, was born.

During my pregnancy I discovered a new side to Phil's character, although it was one that I would have guessed would be there.

He had no time for cramps or cravings.

When I displayed a craving for a certain kind of food, he insisted, "You are quite normal. And you will be quite normal for the length of your pregnancy. Let's get that straight from the start. I will not tolerate any histrionics."

I had a genuine fear of frogs that became worse when I was pregnant. Many frogs lived in our garden and I was afraid that they would jump at me when I opened the garage door.

I pleaded with Phil to open and close the garage door for me, even though I had always done so before.

His reply was predictable.

"Nonsense. Why should you be afraid of frogs? Get this ridiculous attitude out of your head."

The thought of coming home at night terrified me. I knew that I would have to open the garage door.

Fear of frogs was the only obsession I had while I was pregnant. Phil nipped all the others in the bud. He had seen too many women who had become neurotic while they were pregnant and he was determined I would not become that kind of woman.

Later in our married life Phil was to say he was sorry for his approach. He said he might have been too strict during the early years of our married life. Nevertheless, I felt I learned a lot from those experiences.

He cured me of weaknesses I might have had. He stopped any tendencies I might have had to resort to histrionics when they were uncalled for.

I learned to take troubles in my stride through having lived with someone who believed that life was there to be faced—and to be conquered. You cannot lie down and die when troubles overtake you. They have to be stared squarely in the eye and told who is master of the situation.

Phil and I moved to Woodstock, a suburb of Cape Town and close to the central city, in 1939.

Soon Phil's practice started to grow.

We had just got on to our feet again when the news came: War had broken out in Europe. Ten months after he started his new practice, Phil volunteered to join the South African forces and fight in Europe.

There was no question of choice for Phil. Not only did he regard it as his duty to help in the war effort, but, being Jewish, he felt he had to help his own people.

It was a major sacrifice. Phil had moved into rooms that were not equipped for a dental practice. Hot and cold water needed to be provided in addition to the equipment he had carefully chosen and fitted into the room.

As independent as ever, he refused financial help offered by his mother. He wanted to take pride in building a practice of his own, with his own efforts. Now he was forced to sell it all.

In a sense, Phil's actions were part of the secret behind our happiness. When life is easy, you do not need each other as much. But in times of trouble you cling more closely to one another because you have a common enemy. Love becomes meaningful and deep when it is placed in the right perspective.

We knew that in the midst of the fiercest trouble, solace was an arm's length away. That is, until the war ripped us thousands of miles apart.

But I did not let it do so without a fight. Harris and I followed Phil for as long as we could. We kept as close to him as possible during his training period before he finally went into the war zone and it became impossible for us to leave our country.

Phil went to a training camp at Sonderwater in South Africa for a few months before being stationed in Johannesburg, where Harris and I joined him.

He automatically held an officer's rank, being in the medical corps. But, as a lieutenant, Phil felt unworthy of the rank. Men whom he regarded as equals in civilian life were suddenly called upon to salute him. Such a person was my brother-in-law, who was an orderly in the dental unit. He was made a sergeant and had to respect Phil as a superior officer. But in off-duty hours Phil's rank became something of a joke between them.

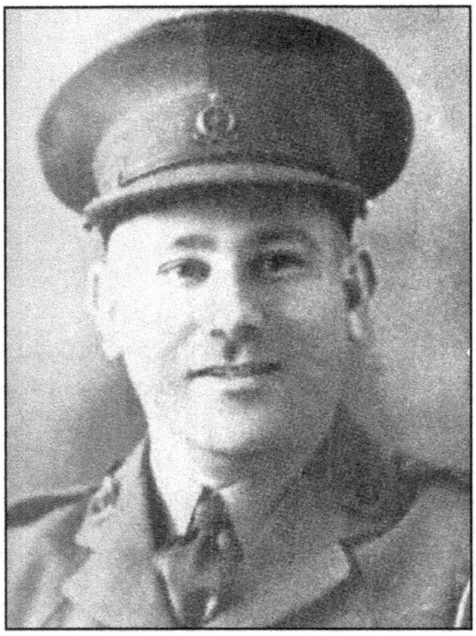

Phil in military uniform

In fact, Phil never became used to being on what was really an artificially higher level. Some took their rank seriously and, inevitably, it went to their heads. Endowed with new powers, they felt they had to use those powers in some way. But Phil did not let that happen to him. He treated the whole thing as a rather ridiculous situation.

One morning, while in training at Sonderwater, the men were awakened by sharp thunderous noises accompanied by rifle fire. Although far off from the war zone, the men were prepared for anything and it was not long before they were all in the dugouts—except one man, who remained in his bed in the tent. The recalcitrant one was Philip Blaiberg.

"Aren't you coming?" called the men.

"No," replied Phil, true to character. "If I'm to be killed, I might as well be killed right here in my warm, comfortable bed."

It turned out it was a mock battle to prepare the men for what was to follow later in the north.

That attitude was Phil's attitude to life generally. He had a fatalistic view. But that fatalism was bonded with a strong belief in his own ability. Fatalistic he certainly was when faced with forces beyond his power to alter. But when he was called upon to fight Phil showed a tenacity of purpose and a fearlessness that were remarkable.

In Johannesburg Phil was stationed at a clinic where the soldiers had their teeth examined before making their way up north. I think there were about six dentists there, most of them older than Phil. It was a shock to the others—and, I suspect, to Phil, too—when he was chosen from this group to go to another training camp at Barberton as an officer in command of the dental unit there.

Phil did not regard it as a promotion, but merely as a new post. This surprised the others, who were all the more ruffled by his matter-of-fact view towards the move.

Harris and I followed Phil to Barberton and he would visit us as often as he could in the hotel in which we stayed.

The men who served with Phil seemed to treat him as a father confessor, even though he was a lot younger than many of them. This approach took place in his practice, too. Phil seemed to engender confidence. People would go to him because they knew he would understand and would be able to advise them.

I remember one man who said that he always felt so safe with Phil around. Phil was a big, strapping fellow so that this man felt protected by his presence. But at the same time his size did not engender fear.

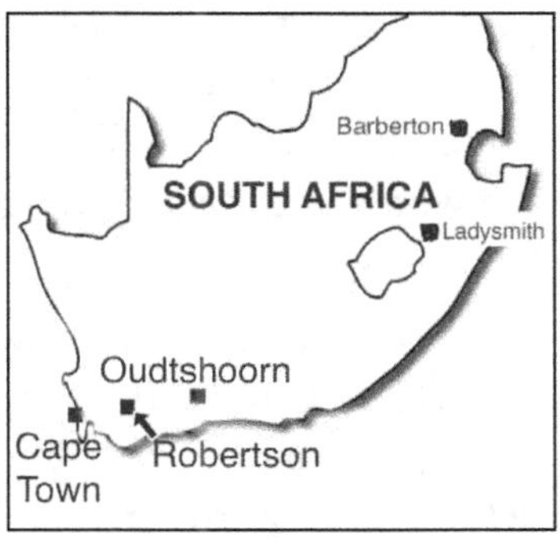

From Barberton we went to Ladysmith in Natal where Phil was transferred. Eventually the time came for Phil to go closer to the scene of the action. He first served in Egypt and then moved to Italy, where he had his own dental unit.

Harris and I did not follow him there, of course. But in a sense we did.

The reason: Phil had a photograph of Harris and me tucked into the lining of his cap. There it served duty as a guard against temptation.

Phil told me when he returned that he would often see an attractive woman and, being a man, certain thoughts would pass through his mind. But quickly he would take off his cap, look at the photograph and think: "Look at those two beautiful things waiting faithfully for me at home.

How can I do anything wrong?"

Back would go his cap on his head and the woman got no more than perhaps another last glance from Phil.

"You were my watchdog in my cap," he told me.

Phil wrote to me often during the war years. I carefully kept every letter. Wherever we moved after his return, I took the letters with me in a trunk.

When in 1966 we moved to our Wynberg flat in Cape Town I was quite prepared to take them with me once more. But when Phil saw them he did not think it would be a good idea. "Really, Eileen. Isn't it time you grew up and got rid of those old letters?"

For 25 years I had carried them around with me. With great reluctance I agreed with Phil. We were moving to a smaller place and there would not be room for all the letters. Little did I realise how valuable the letters would have been later.

As I tore up each letter, I read them again and the memories of those war years flooded back with each word. Although we had been married for eight years at the time, Phil's letters were worthy of a newly-wed.

Every one was a love letter. It did my heart good to consider that it was possible to write like that after being married for so long. By then most couples take one another for granted. Writing a love letter seems pointless and childish to many. But Phil, who would not have pampered me with soft words and sweet nothings while he was close to me, realised that when he was away that was what I needed, in small doses.

Such a separation as the war enforced on us is a severe test. It is a make-or-break test, and if the couple can return to each other after such a test, pick up the threads of their marriage and find there is more love even than before, surely nothing short of death can break such a partnership.

Such was our experience. I lived in Port Elizabeth while Phil was in the army and that was where I waited for him when he returned. I was shocked when I learned of the change the war had made on his outlook on life.

This change came home to me on the first day after he arrived home. My sister prepared a big welcome home party for him the night after he arrived. But Phil was not impressed.

She invited close on 200 people. Phil was not even interested.

"It makes me sick to think that you have gone on living the same sort of lives here while others are starving to death," he said. "Look at that food. Does it not worry you? Others are living in misery and squalour. Is it of no concern to you?"

He was almost nauseated by the sight of the food spread out for the guests. I explained to him that it was a lot to ask of people to change when they had not experienced the horror of war, when they had not watched the grim devices of war, when they had not breathed the stench of war. War cannot be imagined.

Phil tried to understand, but it was some months before he accepted the occasional luxuries which are, to us, a part of normal living. The horror of war left its stamp on his mind and it never quite left him. He avoided parties. Phil was quieter, more deeply mature. For a long time it was more deeply disturbing—torturing, he said.

He was bitter, cynical and disillusioned. How people could laugh, sing and play when others were suffering puzzled him.

"Please, Phil," I would plead. "You cannot change the world. I know you have seen some terrible things, have lived close to the devastation of war. But you must try to forget that now. To me it is revolting.

"We had blackouts while you were away. We could buy petrol only with coupons. We suffered, too."

"Nothing like I saw people suffer." he replied. "Men are murdered—and you celebrate."

"No, Phil, it is not like that. We cannot bear others' burdens forever."

And so the discussions would develop into arguments. He was more sulky than I had known him before. This was not the Phil Blaiberg who would stride out to meet life, prepared for all it could throw in his face. Suddenly, it seemed, life had thrown too much at him. Phil had ducked. Not that Phil himself had been hurt. But he felt so much for others that when he saw them suffer he felt pain in sympathy.

Mere physical pain Phil could have endured, I am sure of that. But to see others take knock after knock dealt out by life made him ponder whether goodness and justice and love had all been buried forever. And a little of him had been buried with them. Slowly the disillusionment was replaced. Like new flesh over an ugly wound, a positive view began to hide his bitterness. But it was always there, like an itch under the skin, to remind him.

Another source of bitterness to Phil at this time was his feelings about those who had not joined up in the armed forces. He had no time for men who had not done their duty, and he made no bones about it. He was particularly bitter about men in his own profession, young men who had moved from the country areas into the towns while the other dentists were fighting and had taken over their practices.

When the war ended, those who had done their duty returned to find their patients going to other dentists. Starting up a new practice again under those circumstances was not easy. That was something criminal to him, and it was many years before he got it out of his head. Jews, particularly, he thought should have joined up without any thought of their families or their reputations.

I saw his point of view and was prone to agree with him. But I felt these obsessions were changing the Philip Blaiberg I knew.

"You cannot go around preaching to others, telling them what they should have done," I told him. "You cannot be angry with people for not thinking the same things as you do."

He was obstinate, as I have told you, and would not be tolerant of other points of view in this regard. As time went on, however, he became more understanding and more tolerant.

Indeed, I believe this whole experience matured him. For example, before the war we had our own ideas of religion and what one should believe and these led to strong disagreements at times, after the war we were more prepared to tolerate the other person's point of view.

I believe the war did a lot to help Phil to change in that respect and we developed a philosophy of agreeing to disagree. Occasions on which I had to be the one to give in for the sake of peace became less.

Certainly we found that a man and a woman do not have to think alike to be an ideally married couple.

To assist ex-servicemen to get going again in their practices as doctors or dentists, a number of other ex-servicemen were allotted to them so that they would have a nucleus of patients with which to start. Phil also received such a nucleus of patients. It is a tribute to him that he kept many of them right until the time he retired. But a big problem that faced him was getting rooms in Cape Town. It seemed to us it would be easier finding gold in the city than suitable rooms for a dentist. What we eventually had to do was buy out an artist, including the paintings. That was the only way we could get accommodation.

Phil was then 33, not an easy age from which to start right from the beginning again. And Harris was already eight at that time.

It was not all that long that the new practice was under way when disillusionment began to show in Phil. His experiences in the war years again caused this. It was only a year since his return to civilian life that he said to me one day: "Eileen, I just cannot take private practice any longer."

The trouble was that he had become so accustomed to the people he had dealt with in the army that he could no longer tolerate the petty foibles of his daily patients. Phil was the last person to worry about a bedside manner. He had learned not to pander to people while in the army and when he returned to the small, vain worries of the city dwellers he tended to become impatient.

He liked straight talk. He liked to tell people the truth.

One of his biggest bugbears were those whom he liked to call "the society ladies". Granted every dentist has his fair share of these type of people, but Phil could not forget the war and the men he had met through it. He had many of them as his patients, and it was this nucleus that he regarded as his finest clients.

"They come to have their teeth pulled or to have dentures fitted and they expect to walk out as beauty queens," Phil would say about the "society ladies".

"I would like to say to them: 'Madam, I can change your teeth, but I cannot change your face.'

"No, I can take no more of this. You have to play up to them, nurse them. My patience is coming to an end."

There was an exception, however, among the ex-servicemen. One of them had received a medal for bravery and yet when he had to come and see Phil to have his teeth examined, he was as frightened as a little child.

"What's wrong with you?" Phil asked a man one day as he worked on his teeth, which were in a terrible state.

"You are shaking. Your nerves are shot."

The man looked up at Phil. "Doctor, I would rather go into a minefield than to have an injection to have a filling."

Those were the sort of people with whom Phil could work. He knew that man was genuinely brave for he had seen what he had done in the war. So he talked him into having less fear of going to the dentist.

When it came to trying to pander to the whims of "society ladies," however, Phil drew the line. "I'm just not made for this kind of life any more," he told me one day. "I'm going to give it up."

"But, Phil, after all our struggling, our looking for rooms."

"No, Eileen, I have made up my mind. Poorer people appreciate when you are trying to help them. Perhaps there I will feel a greater sense of achievement, of satisfaction and fulfillment. Because I am not getting that now."

I was horrified. Surely not another new start. But I knew better than to argue with Phil. If that was how he felt, it was unfortunate, but it would be pointless pushing against him and would merely serve to aggravate matters.

"Where will you work?"

"I am going to work for the City Council. They have started a dental clinic for underprivileged people."

We sold the practice. At least we got back quite a lot of our investment, plus a little compensation for the goodwill he had built up.

Phil was an idealist, however. And, after three years of working at the dental clinic, once again disillusionment began to set in. It was not the sort of work he had imagined it would be. It became routine and impersonal and that sense of fulfillment, that satisfaction that comes from knowing you are serving your fellowman still eluded him.

It was as though they were punching holes in computer cards and he was pulling teeth. He was too great an idealist to regard this as the fruit of a high calling.

Work at the dental clinic finally came to an end when Phil contracted what is called a "dentist's elbow" that came from doing too many extractions daily. That helped him to make the decision that, in any event, he had come close to making. It was the last straw that broke the camel's back. So, after three years, it was once again back to square one.

This time Phil chose to start his new practice in the Cape Town suburb of Goodwood. He saw this area was growing and many new people were moving into it. Each time he started a practice I would work as his nurse for the first few months and when he started at Goodwood it was no exception.

By this time we had moved into a new house in Weltevreden Avenue, Rondebosch—a house we were to occupy for 21 years. We had lived in hotels before that—and I had lived in hotels for so much of my life.

My mother-in-law said she would lend us some money to get our own house.

We shopped around and attended a number of auction sales. Finally along came the house in Weltevreden Avenue.

Phil did not even look at the house when I told him how impressed I was with it. "If you like it", he said, "that is a good enough recommendation for me."

I went to the auction sale. The house had been neglected outside and so went for far less than it should have. I regarded the neglect as a challenge, however, and it was not long before I had the garden trimmed and flower-filled.

We received a lot of pleasure out of that house and I still associate it with most of the happiness of our married life.

While we were there, and just as Phil was getting his Goodwood practice going, our second child, Jill, was born, nine years after Harris's birth.

About this time, Phil took a holiday for a month. It was one of the few holidays he took. He worked as hard as anyone I have ever known.

He worked always for us, increased his life insurance coverage, too, determined that we should have no worries should he die. "Enjoy yourself while you can. Let us go on holiday and spend the money you are earning in that way so that you, too, will be able to feel the benefit of it.

"I cannot enjoy life unless I know you and the children are provided for, Eileen."

That was typical of Phil, always caring about us and not putting himself first. I thought he was being silly then, but I must admit that today I appreciate his foresight and realise that without the insurance Jill and I would not be able to relax as we could. Money would have been a constant worry.

Those days were among the happiest of our married lives. There was no hint of the troubles to come. It seemed as though we did not have a care in the world. After Phil had been in Goodwood for some years, he received a telephone call from the dentist who had bought his Cape Town practice at the time Phil went to work for the dental clinic. He asked him whether he would not like to buy it back again. The man was a British immigrant and had decided to return to London.

Phil was thrilled. He just could not wait to get back into his old practice again. Many of the people who live in Goodwood are Afrikaans-speaking. As a result Phil had many patients who spoke that language. This was no problem to him, for he spoke Afrikaans as a young boy and grew up with the language. In fact, it was his home language until he was nine.

As a result there was never any question of ethnic bias in Phil's practice, particularly in Goodwood, but in fact wherever he was. He loved everybody and they loved him and the widespread nature of his practice when he retired was proof of that; Afrikaans-speaking, English-speaking, Jews, regardless.

6

Six years after Phil's first heart attack in 1955, which I described at the start of this book, the next major shock hit us. On August 2, 1961, our son Harris died.

Although Phil recovered from his heart attack, he never seemed to recover from the death of his son—his greatest friend on earth.

Life was meaningless to us immediately after Harris's death. We groped aimlessly to deduct sense from what was happening around us. Like two people suddenly stricken with blindness we felt surrounded by a blackness as deep as death itself.

At first, it seemed, the darkness had descended right between us, cutting us off from one another, too.

Phil was introspective, quiet, almost withdrawn from reality. Yet as we groped we found each other.

For a full year we withdrew into our shells, satisfied to let the world drift past us in a bouncy bubbling stream as we sat and sobbed on the bank.

No other single experience in my life has ever matched that time of sorrow. Yet, in a sense, I look back to see this as a grim rehearsal for testing times of sorrow in the future—sorrow aplenty that was to come.

I am amazed that today I can think about that event without that heart-rending hollow feeling that tore through my insides at that time and choked me in tears before I could continue to discuss it.

A part of you dies when you lose a child. Phil compared it to his coronary.

"The wound heals eventually, but the scar remains forever." Both scars remained forever with Phil. The scar of his coronary stayed on his weakened heart and the scar of Harris's death left its imprint on his mind. It took us years to recover.

It seems difficult to believe, but it was more than five years after Harris had died that we danced again. We were at a wedding on March 5, 1967. We decided almost simultaneously that we would throw aside our troubles and make the most of living again.

Our daughter Jill looked so radiantly beautiful that night. We looked at her and we realised we had so much to be thankful for as we whirled together across the floor. It seemed that dawn was peeping over the hills, telling us the long darkness was over.

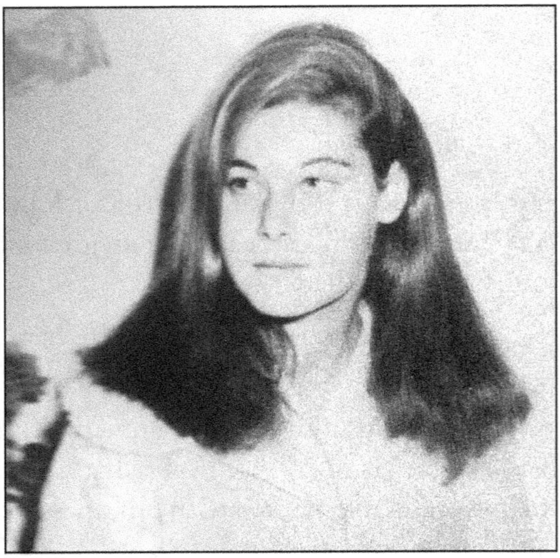

Jill Blaiberg, 19

But it was not. Our joy was short-lived. Those few carefree hours were merely a prelude to the sombre drama that was to occupy our lives for many months to come.

7

Towards the end of October, 1968, Phil became so seriously ill that he gave up all hope of recovery without an operation of some sort.

Most days he did not have the energy to get out of bed. Daily his will to fight was being eaten away by his failing strength. When Phil reached the stage where he felt it was useless to fight you knew he felt the end was near.

"If only they would do something," he said. "It must either be an operation or death. I know I'm getting worse and worse. I cannot go on like this any longer.

"I am going to speak to Professor Velva Schrire (a leading Cape Town cardiologist) and insist that I have an operation. They can experiment on me if they like. I don't care any longer.

"Do they think I am going to hang around here at home indefinitely? No, it's an operation or death.

"It's do or die."

Phil spoke to Professor Schrire, who pacified him, saying: "We will see."

That month of November was almost hell. Phil could scarcely breathe and it was agony watching him try. I wondered how a man could go on like that, trying to live, but knowing all the time that no matter how hard he tried death was slowly gaining the upper hand.

By December 2, he was virtually bedridden, getting up only occasionally.

I will never forget the events of those two days. They started on the afternoon of Saturday, December 2. Phil was not looking at all well. I was extremely concerned.

I telephoned our house doctor, Dr. Kohn, and asked him to get in touch with Professor Schrire.

"Maybe he can see to it that Phil gets put into the hospital," I said.

Dr. Kohn promised to do his best.

By a series of coincidences, I was out that Saturday evening. It was one of the few times I left Phil on his own, although our domestic servant Katie was there. Dr. Kohn had telephoned the apartment, but did not want to worry me when he was told I was visiting my brother.

The next morning I tried to telephone Dr. Kohn when I received his message. But he was playing golf. I telephoned the golf club. They assured me they would ask Dr. Kohn to telephone me as soon as he left the course.

Then came lunchtime on Sunday, December 3.

Phil's voice had been getting softer and softer. It was an effort for him to talk, even when he wanted to say something important. But that day a strong voice shouted to me from his bedroom as I was preparing lunch in the kitchen.

"Eileen!"

What was it? Was he in trouble? No, his voice sounded too excited for that. Something had happened to make him suddenly happy. What could it be?

"Eileen, come and listen to this. Come and hear what has happened. It's the most fantastic thing. And right here in South Africa.

"What Phil? What has happened?"

"A man has been given a new heart."

"That's wonderful." It was, of course, the news of the world's first heart transplant operation on Louis Washkansky that Phil had heard on the radio. But the significance did not register with me at first.

"What a lucky man," Phil said, still enthusiastic more than I thought he was able to be in his state of health.

"But, even more than that, can you imagine what this will do for this country?"

The news that day alone did wonders for Phil. He had lost a lot of interest in life. Now suddenly there was meaning in what was happening around him. The flame of hope had been lit. In fact, Phil's awakened enthusiasm for life held more excitement to me than the announcement of the heart transplant operation. As I thought about the momentous event, however, I pondered what it could mean in our lives if only...

But, no, I said to myself, don't hope, don't think of it. Phil's too ill.

Oh, how lucky some people can be.

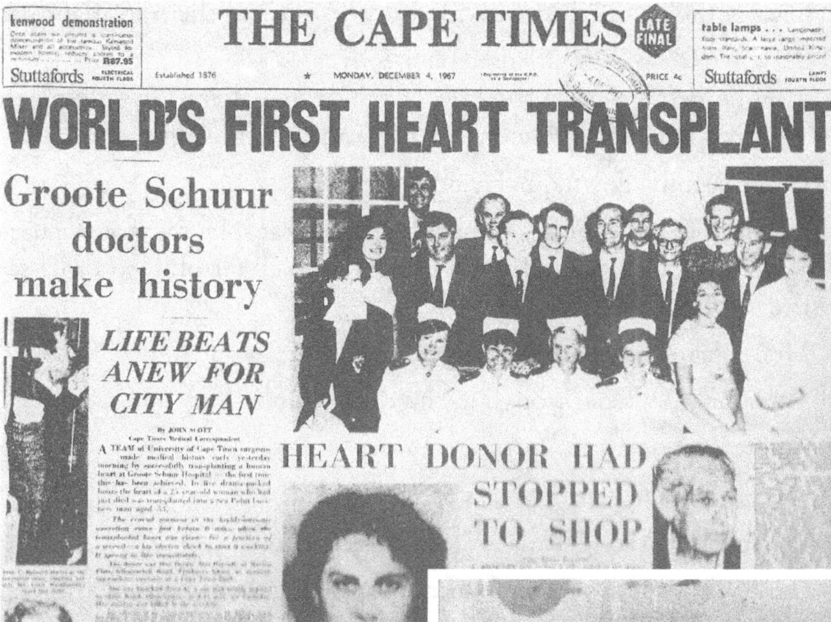

kenwood demonstration

Stuttafords

THE CAPE TIMES LATE FINAL

table lamps . . .

Stuttafords

Established 1876 ★ MONDAY, DECEMBER 4, 1967 PRICE 4c

WORLD'S FIRST HEART TRANSPLANT

Groote Schuur doctors make history

LIFE BEATS ANEW FOR CITY MAN

By JOHN SCOTT

Cape Times Medical Correspondent

HEART DONOR HAD STOPPED TO SHOP

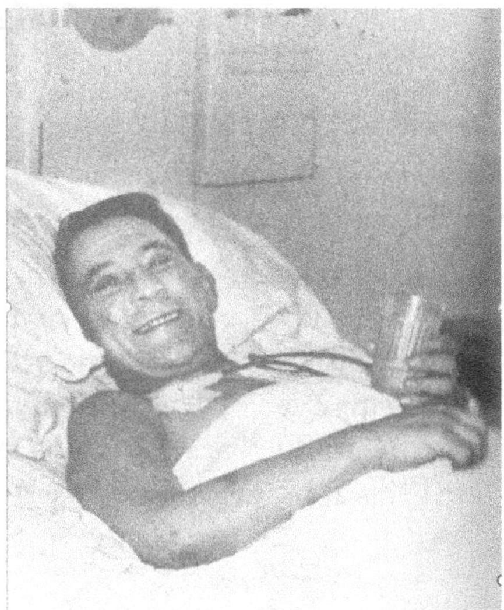

Louis Washkansky

It was a busy afternoon, as most Sunday afternoons had come to be. Friends came to ask whether they could take Phil for a drive or they came just to visit him. That afternoon we had even more visitors than usual. But I asked them not to worry Phil. He was, after all, extremely ill and he was too weary to speak to a lot of people. I spent the afternoon moving back and forth from the lounge (to see if our visitors were happy) to Phil (to see whether he was alright).

When I went into his room at about 4 p.m. Phil looked blue and worse than ever.

"No," I thought, "I cannot bear this another day."

Phil, too, was reaching the end of his tether.

"I cannot go on living like this anymore, please ask them to do something for me."

Clearly the stimulation provided by the news of the transplant had dissipated already.

I was desperate when I saw how ill he was that afternoon—desperate for any straw at which to clutch, any hope anyone could give me.

Phil was going down quickly now.

I went to the telephone. Perhaps the heart transplant was at the back of my mind—that was a straw at which to clutch. I telephoned Professor Schrire direct.

Mrs. Schrire answered the telephone.

Thoughts tumbled through my muddled mind.

"I'm terribly sorry to worry you Ruth."

"Not at all. Val's dying to talk to you."

"I just want to congratulate the heart team on..."

"Hullo, Eileen," Professor Schrire said, taking the telephone from his wife. "Did you telephone me about the proposition?"

"What proposition?"

"Didn't your doctor tell you I telephoned to say that Phil is going to be the next transplant recipient."

I often wonder what I would have thought then had I not heard about the Washkansky transplant—and I might well have heard about "the proposition" the previous day had the series of coincidences not led to my missing it. As it was, I heard afterwards that Dr. Kohn had not taken Professor Schrire all that seriously when he told him about the suggestion; he also had not heard yet about the Washkansky transplant.

"Val, I cannot believe it. This is the most superb news I have ever heard."

"Are you pleased?"

"I am absolutely thrilled. But how do I break the news to Phil?"

"You will find a way."

"When can I bring him in?"

"I will tell you. But don't let the newspapers or anybody else know, because this is one time we are going to do it quietly and nobody is going to know about it."

I ran in and told our visitors, but I asked them not to tell the newspapers. I did not know at that stage what a futile hope it was that the news would not reach the ears of the press.

My visitors were not as impressed as I was. Quite the contrary.

"What are you so excited about?" they asked.

"I don't suppose you can understand my excitement. Your husbands are not dying," I said.

"For the first time in nine months I have been given a little hope. You don't understand what this means to me. The past nine months have been filled with despair, with waning hope. Now there is hope at last."

I could see nothing but success ahead. After all, Washkansky was still alive.

But one big hurdle still lay ahead. I had to break the news to Phil. My problem here was that I was still trying to make out to him that he was not as bad as he thought. Each time he complained or slipped into despair I would try to boost his morale by saying he would soon get better. Now suddenly I was going to tell him that his heart was so rotten that he was going to get a new one. I had to change character in the middle of the act.

The mere change was not the important part, however. What was important was the effect that this would have on Phil's thinking.

After all, he knew I had been talking to the doctors, who would presumably have told me the truth. And so while I continued to be confident that he would improve, he could gain hope from my confidence, even though he realised he was getting weaker.

Should I tell him, however, of the heart transplant decision, I was afraid he would realise that I had been play-acting in the past. And he would realise how bad his condition really was. Would that not have a bad effect on his heart?

These thoughts were in my dazed mind as I went through the formalities of entertaining our guests. They finally left at 5 p.m. Then the time came to go into Phil's room. But the problem was still unsolved. What was I going to say to him?

The problem was solved for me, however. At 5:30 p.m., while I was with him in the room, Phil suddenly took a turn for the worse.

"Eileen, I cannot go on like this."

He was deathly white. He battled to breathe.

"Telephone Professor Schrire. Tell him to do something."

Phil struggled to speak. But the words came to me spontaneously. "Phil, what would you say if they offered you a new heart?"

"Please, Eileen, please. Don't fool around with my feelings. You know I am not lucky enough to get a chance like that."

"But darling you are."

His face sparkled into life. Suddenly he could breathe more easily.

"Tell me more, tell me more."

I told him of the conversation with Professor Schrire.

"How do you feel?" I asked.

He stretched out his hands.

"Just take me as quickly as possible. Let them give me a new heart and I will be the happiest man in the world."

I put my arms around him and we laughed and cried in a crazy mixture of joy and confused fear.

Then in the middle of it all, he asked: "Why are you so happy about it? You are the one who has been saying I am getting better."

I looked him straight in the eye. No acting, no back-turning now.

"I am going to put all my cards on the table, Phil. For the first time since your heart attack I am going to tell you the honest truth.

"I have known from the word go that there was no hope for you. There was nothing they could do for you. Can you imagine what it means to me now to think that I might have my husband for a little longer?

"I didn't expect you to live for even as long as you have lived because you have been getting so bad."

He looked at me in surprised admiration.

"You are a fabulous person, Eileen. But more than that you are a wonderful actress. You deserve an Oscar. I think we will make you the film star of the year.

"I can swear to you, never did it enter my mind that you knew a thing because you acted so happily and brightly. I knew you were terribly worried, but...

"I cannot tell you what you have done for me. To think that you lived for nine months without showing the trouble you have been through."

There were few moments in our lives when we were closer to one another than then. A minute of revelation and the bonds that linked us were drawn more tightly than ever before.

We both realised how much we meant to each other and how important it was that we have as much time together as could be spared to us.

As I crawled into the same double bed again that evening, we marvelled at our love for one another. We realised our love was deep and powerful, for we both had been acting unnatural lives for fear of hurting the other.

He had realised in the past three months that he had been fading fast. Yet he had not wanted to be blunt about it, although at the same time he saw the need to be realistic. Not wanting to upset me, he had tried to couch the facts he knew in euphemistic terms.

That night the strain of nine months was suddenly broken. I felt an immense calm, in spite of Phil's condition.

All our married lives we had always told one another everything, but for nine tense months we had tried to act unnatural parts. Now that was gone, wiped away in an instant. In addition, there was reason for hope. A new heart was waiting somewhere for Phil and there was no need any longer to live a lie.

I awoke the following morning to a new world. Now there was hope. The symbol of our joy lay in Cape Town's Groote Schuur Hospital registering beep...beep...beep on a monitor.

Each day, we read and listened to every word on Louis Washkansky. As the reports came through—"He is doing well"—our happiness increased.

It was difficult waiting after that.

A few days passed and I telephoned Professor Schrire.

"When are you going to operate?"

"Eileen, have a little patience. The whole heart team is still busy looking after Louis Washkansky.

"You must wait for him to be discharged and well on the way to recovery before we undertake your husband's operation. Just keep your husband happy and well."

I had a certain amount of success keeping Phil happy, but keeping him well was not a task I could easily perform.

About eight days after the Washkansky operation Phil started getting seriously ill again.

Professor Schrire must have got to know my voice well in those days. Again I telephoned.

"I don't think we can wait any longer. He is deteriorating fast. If you want to keep him alive you must admit him to the hospital."

"Look, Eileen, I will go into the whole thing. I will talk to the doctors and see what we can do."

He telephoned me back later that day.

"We have a bed for your husband on the 16th—that is in five days time. But remember this. We are doing it on the 16th because that is a public holiday. We are going to get him in as quietly as we can without any fuss. We want no newspapers there."

Other doctors told me: "This must be done in absolute secrecy because this time we are determined we are not going to have the bedlam that we had with Washkansky.

"You just don't know what is going on here at the hospital. We thought it would just be for the first few days, but it is every day and all day.

"They hide in the passages, jump out of corridors, and it is impossible to keep order.

"We are terrified of strangers going so far as to jump into Washkansky's room. There is the great danger of infection. We just need to be very careful and very quiet about all this."

The newspapers heard a couple of days after the Washkansky operation that my husband was going to be next. I believe it was through a process of elimination.

Unfortunately one of the doctors at the hospital let slip that the next person on their list was a dentist. It was their fault. They were the ones who wanted to keep it quiet.

Apparently the newspapers telephoned every dentist in town. Eventually they realised it must be my husband because he was the one who had retired through ill health.

My instructions from the doctors were to deny any knowledge that my husband would be the next recipient. And I kept to those instructions.

A wily reporter found his way around those denials, however. He telephoned Phil, who answered himself. I was out at the time.

"Hullo, Dr. Blaiberg," he said, without introducing himself. "When are you going to have your operation?"

Phil, not suspecting that he was speaking to a reporter, more or less confirmed in the short conversation that followed that he would be the next transplant recipient.

Once his name was published, the telephone calls grew into an avalanche.

Those telephone calls heralded a shattering of the peace in our lives. The curtain of privacy surrounding our lives was torn apart.

Never again would Phil be Dr. Blaiberg, the retired dentist slowly dying of a weak heart.

From now on he was Dr. Philip Blaiberg, South Africa's next heart transplant recipient.

They spoke to us from all over the world, snatching at any news I could give them, no matter how small.

I believe I started getting a bad name among the press at that time because I refused to give interviews or hand out photographs.

I want to explain why it was that I did that. Firstly it was at the specific request of the doctors. They were the ones attending to my husband, they knew what was best for his health, and I followed their advice implicitly.

Secondly we were sickened by the publicity surrounding Louis Washkansky and his family.

I know that Anne Washkansky (with whom I have since become friendly) also hated the publicity that turned the operation into something bordering on a circus.

We thought we would not like to become a comic opera.

We thought what was happening was quite undignified. After all, it was medical history. It should have been done in a quiet dignified way.

In consultation with the doctors, Phil and I had decided that if he had his operation it was not going to be a sensation-mongering affair. It was to be something to save a man's life, not to provide the world's news media with a dramatic story.

After the operation had been performed we would announce it to the world.

8

Two days before Phil was due to be admitted to the hospital he had another attack which was so severe that I thought at one stage that he might never get the chance to undergo the heart transplant operation.

"Call the doctor." he begged. "I don't think I can live. If you can't get hold of Dr. Kohn, call Dr. Getz, but it has got to be within minutes."

Dr. Kohn was attending the graduation of his son who also became a doctor. So I called Dr. Getz who did not take long to get to our house as he lived just across the road.

Dr. Getz said Phil needed oxygen immediately and should be taken to the hospital where it could be administered. As Dr. Getz was attending to my husband, Dr. Kohn came in. He had heard about Phil's attack and had come as soon as he could.

Both agreed it was an emergency. Moments counted and there was no time to waste at all.

Again I telephoned Professor Schrire.

"We cannot wait until the sixteenth," I said. "He is going fast."

"Right, Eileen, an ambulance will be there soon."

The ambulance came and Phil was carefully placed in it. As we went to the hospital, I wondered about Professor Schrire's warning about the press. Already I had experienced their ability to ferret out information. Was it possible that they had found out about Phil's admission today?

My fears were groundless. Phil could have been any patient as far as the press was concerned. It was late in the afternoon as he entered ward D-1. The hospital staff administered oxygen immediately. I, too, breathed more easily as I saw Phil doing so. The doctors gave him injections. I could see he was in safe hands and my worries eased slightly.

Anxious days were to follow, days in which our faith in the transplant was to be tested.

Every day was a new battle to keep Phil going. He seemed to be teetering on the very edge of death. But somehow he succeeded in keeping from falling and at times he even managed to speak a little.

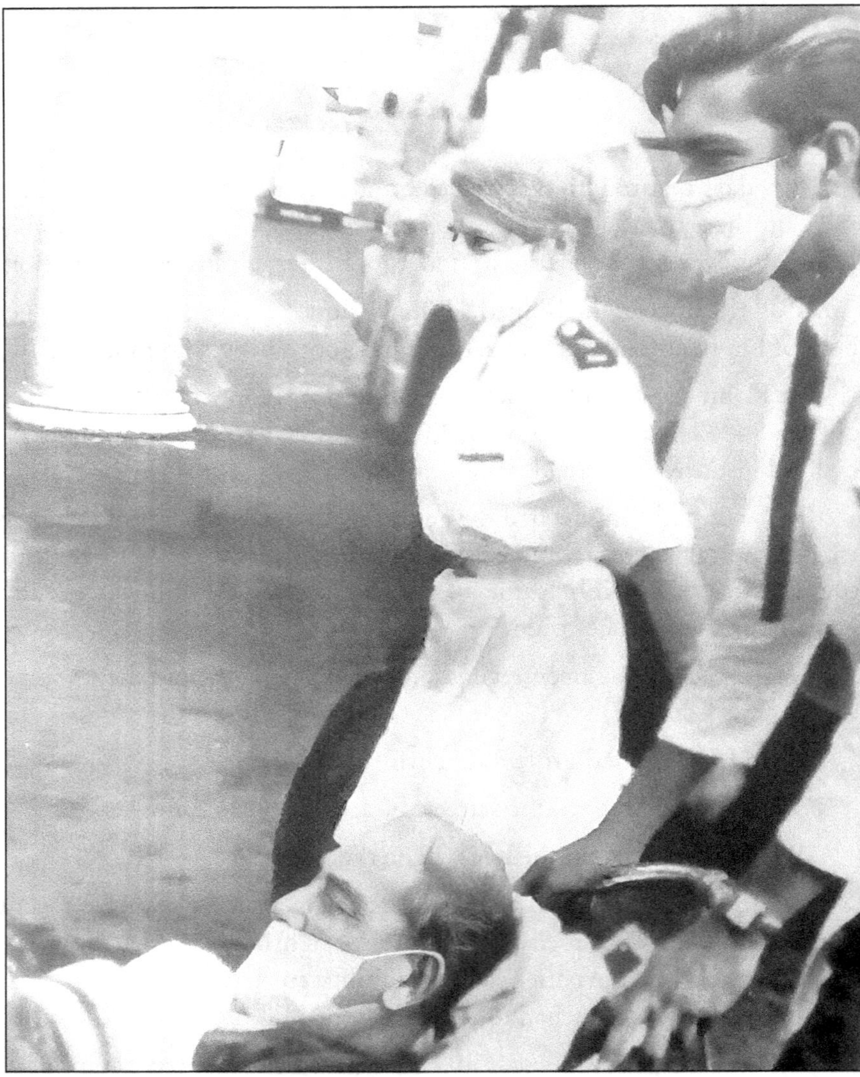

Phil entering the hospital

"I don't know when they are going to do this operation," he kept saying. "I wonder if they will ever do it in time?"

He had been in hospital for about five days when he told me he had met members of the heart team.

"What a fabulous crowd they are. They came in one by one today to meet me and they all said: 'Boy, are we keen to get stuck into you, Dr. Blaiberg. Dentists have always hurt us, now we can get our own back.'

They assured me, however, I would be fine."

One day he was really excited.

"Guess who I met this morning?" he said. "Professor Barnard. And what an experience that was. I was half-drugged and I felt so sleepy.

"Then I woke up and saw a man at the end of my bed. I didn't know whether I was dreaming or even if it was real, but he looked so much like Christ to me.

"A beautiful man, with such aesthetic features.

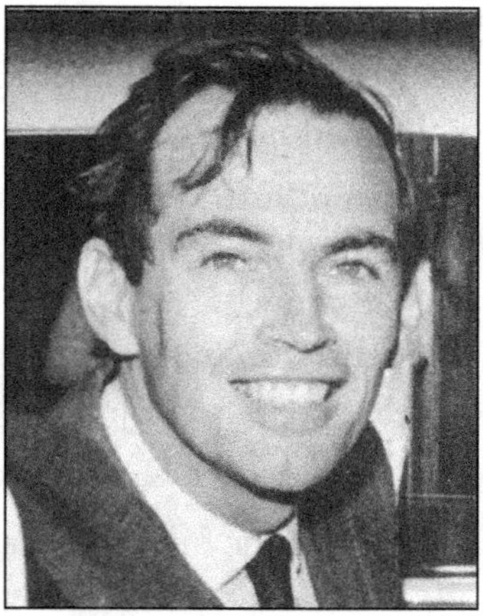
Chris Barnard

"Then I looked again. And I thought he looked so much like South African prime minister General Smuts looked in his youth.

"The man said, in rather an Afrikaans accent: 'Dr. Blaiberg, do you know who I am?' I felt terrible, because I realised this was somebody I should know and still was not sure whether I was awake. Then I blinked and I looked again and I said: 'I am so sorry, but I do not recognise you.'

"Then I looked at his hands. And I thought: What beautiful hands. Then he said: 'I am Professor Barnard.'

"'I am so sorry, I should have recognised you from the photographs I have seen of you,' I said. 'But I want to tell you that you are more impressive than the photographs.'"

Strangely enough these impressions were a lot different from those of Mrs. Washkansky who told me when I got to know her later that her first impressions of Professor Barnard were: "This child, how can he do such a big operation on my husband?"

Phil's reaction surprised me, particularly because he was not the type of man who is easily impressed. He usually got to know the person before he liked them, then once he was your friend he was your friend for life. He was too deep a person to take instant likes or dislikes.

During this time I had the difficult problem of breaking the news of the proposed transplant to Jill in Israel. It was not going to be easy to sit down and write to our only child and tell her that her father was going to have his old heart cut out and a new one stitched in its place. It is far preferable to explain something like this first hand, when you can watch the reaction of the person to whom you are talking, when you can see their eyes and alter your approach if necessary. Writing a letter is impersonal.

Alone in a strange country, she was to hear that her father was going to undergo an entirely new operation. I thought she would be confused and would find it tough to deal with what was happening.

After giving the matter much thought, I wrote Jill a long letter. I told her of the wonderful operation that had been performed on Louis Washkansky and how it was the first of its sort in the world.

I went into a lot of detail, enclosing newspaper cuttings. This letter was intended to prepare Jill for what was to follow. I thought it better to let her know my attitude to the operation, then I would follow this with another letter telling her that her father was deteriorating.

Gradually, I would educate her about the transplant, cushion the blow, wait a week or two, then break the news to her.

I wrote the first letter and waited patiently for her reply. Phil had told me that, although he knew he was seriously ill, under no circumstances was I to write in such a way as to bring Jill back.

"Whatever happens to me—even if something goes wrong with the transplant, please don't bring her back, Eileen," he said. "She will return when she is finished with her course."

Jill had ended her stay at a kibbutz and was studying Hebrew. Phil knew that if Jill came back then it would interfere with her studies and spoil her plans for the future.

I was priding myself on the good piece of spade work I had done in my letter to Jill when a friend of Jill's, who lives in Cape Town, telephoned me to say that she had heard a radio report that Jill had heard for the first time that her father was going to undergo a heart transplant.

Shocked that she had to hear it in another way, I quickly telephoned the South African Broadcasting Corporation to check whether she had heard correctly. They kindly said they would get the original report by telex from Johannesburg, where it had emanated.

About half-an-hour later the SABC telephoned me back. They said the report showed an Israeli journalist had visited Jill to ask her how she felt about the news that her father was to have a transplant.

Jill was understandably upset at hearing the news in that way. She must have wondered why I had said nothing about it in my letters, but she quickly recovered her composure and told the journalist that, whatever happened, she had confidence in Professor Barnard and in South Africa. I was proud to think that she had handled the press so well in what was her first taste of being in the news spotlight.

But my pride in Jill was overshadowed that day by my sense of failure in not having told her sooner. Certainly, I had done what I thought best, placing Jill's feelings above everything else.

I had calculated without taking the news media into consideration, however—a bitter mistake that I was to try to avoid with all my power in the future.

I telephoned Jill in Israel, but I could not hear what she was saying. My frustration grew. I wrote a letter explaining all that the heart team was doing and planned to do.

"Your father is pleased about the operation," I wrote. "You shouldn't worry, I will let you know when the operation is due."

Jill replied she was unhappy about what the press was doing to her. This unsophisticated girl of 20 was suddenly besieged from all sides by the world's press.

Whereas I had only the local press to contend with, Jill was inundated with journalists from many places outside Israel who flew in to speak to her.

An English journalist later told me the newspaper offices received a cable saying Dr. Blaiberg's daughter was beautiful. This was too good for any self-respecting journalist to miss.

Not only was Jill the daughter of the world's next heart transplant recipient—an outstanding story in itself—but also was attractive.

These two facts added up to the best story in some time—and they jumped on it.

As the news-seekers flew in droves into Israel, Jill could at first not cope with this strange, unnerving experience.

She ran away from them because she had always shunned publicity. They would come at all times. When she was eating, others in the communal dining room would warn her there was someone at the door who wanted to see her and Jill would flee to the safety of her bedroom. There she would stay for hours, frightened to come out; there could have been a newsman outside.

Soon not even the privacy of her bedroom was respected by the newsmen hungry for a story they had to get at all costs. They opened her bedroom door without knocking and took photographs of her in bed or in her gown. No privacy was left to her at any time. Wherever she went she felt hunted.

Eventually the news hunters wore her down so much that there was only one way out—to give in. So she condescended to interviews and all across the world television viewers saw a quiet 20-year-old speak confidently of her father and her country.

Phil and I closely followed Louis Washkansky' progress. Was he not the symbol of life to us? As long as the new heart was still beating in his chest so did our hope for the future. He was a living example of what the doctors would do for Phil.

The first hint that all was not going well with Washkansky came shortly after Phil had been admitted to the hospital. I tried not to let it disturb me.

I had great confidence in the heart team and I was sure they would see that Washkansky pulled through. Yet one must accept the facts, not your twisted interpretation of them.

The fact was that Washkansky was slipping.

The torment of those days was terrifyingly real to us.

Desperately I prayed that Washkansky would live. In the hospital, Phil followed Washkansky' s progress on his portable radio. At home I read every word written on him in the newspapers and eagerly soaked up every word spoken on the air.

Then the doctors said there was no more hope for Washkansky. Where now is your dream, Eileen? It has become a nightmare.

If they cannot save Louis, why should it work for Phil? If he died the operation would have been a failure. Why then, perform another? It would be a flash in the pan.

And that would be that. No more hope, no more dreams. Our little

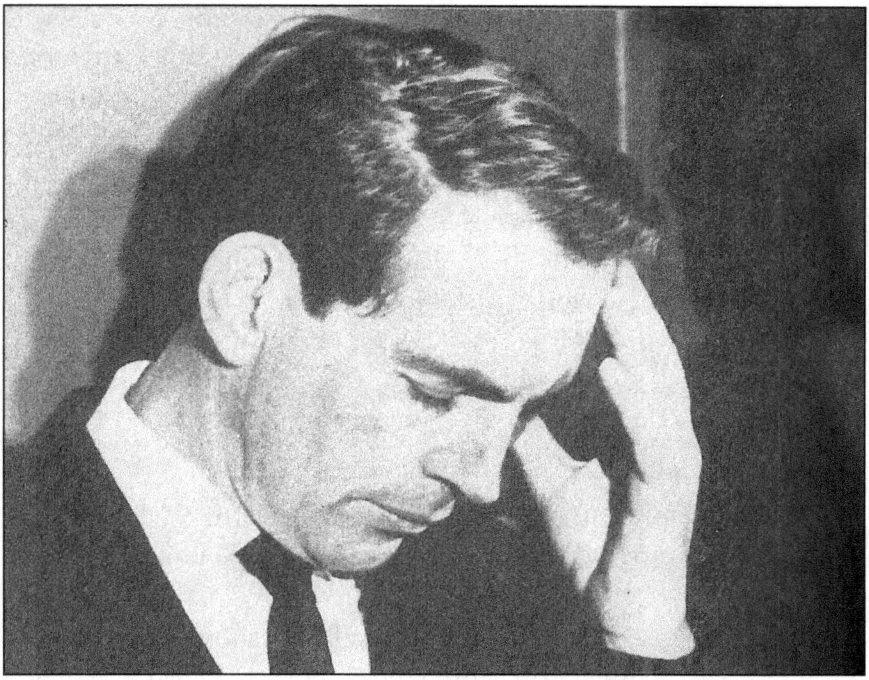

bit of hoped-for heaven would prove to have been a fool's paradise.

My depression became worse as Washkansky lost ground.

Then came the morning of December 22.

"Louis Washkansky is dead."

Our little bit of blue sky was gone. The black clouds had rolled over it again. It was even worse now than before. Why had they ever buoyed up our hopes with the promise of a transplant?

As I dragged myself to work, I knew a little bit of me had died in Groote Schuur Hospital that day. For me, the Cape's carefree summer day was draped with the bleakness of mid-winter.

When my brother saw me he asked, "What can I do to help you?"

"I would like to see Phil, Abe. I would like to know what his reactions are when he hears that Washkansky is gone."

"You cannot go alone. I will telephone my wife. She will take you to see him."

Half-an-hour later we were on our way to Groote Schuur Hospital. I felt as though the events of the past 18 days had been wiped away. Here we are again, back to square one. Back to the depression, back to facing the prospect of Phil's dying soon, back to play-acting again. He must not know the effect that this has had on me. He must still think there is hope, somehow, somewhere. I will have to cheer him even though, God knows, there is little left in me on which to draw.

Somehow I managed to smile as we walked into ward D-1.

"Eileen!" Phil said. "What are you doing here this morning? Aren't you supposed to be at work?"

"The office was not too busy today. I got a lift with Sadie and I thought I would pop in just to say hullo to you."

"Professor Barnard came to see me a little while ago," Phil said. "He said he was coming back soon. Wait here, you'll see him."

He was so pleased to see me that it made me feel worse. I did not know how I was going to bring myself to tell him of Louis Washkansky's death. It was clear he did not yet know the news.

Then I saw a sad, but handsome man walk into the ward. I recognised Professor Barnard immediately from the photographs I had seen of him. I got up to go, thinking Professor Barnard could tell Phil alone. But as I did, Phil introduced me, telling Professor Barnard that I would go out of the room while he talked to him.

"No," Professor Barnard said. "I want to talk to you both. Please don't go."

He was white and drawn. As sorry as I was for myself, I was more sorry for him. He had the responsibility of performing the operation. Now he was left to tell my husband the sad news.

"Dr. Blaiberg, I suppose you've heard Mr. Washkansky died a couple of hours ago," Professor Barnard said.

Phil gasped. "Oh, did he? I couldn't understand why every time I wanted to listen to the radio this morning someone grabbed it away from me."

"Oh, professor, I am so sorry for you," I said. "As sorry as I am for Mrs. Washkansky, I am even more sorry for you and the team. You put so much into the operation. What can I do to help you?"

Professor Barnard turned to Phil.

"Dr. Blaiberg, I feel like a pilot that has crashed. Do you think you

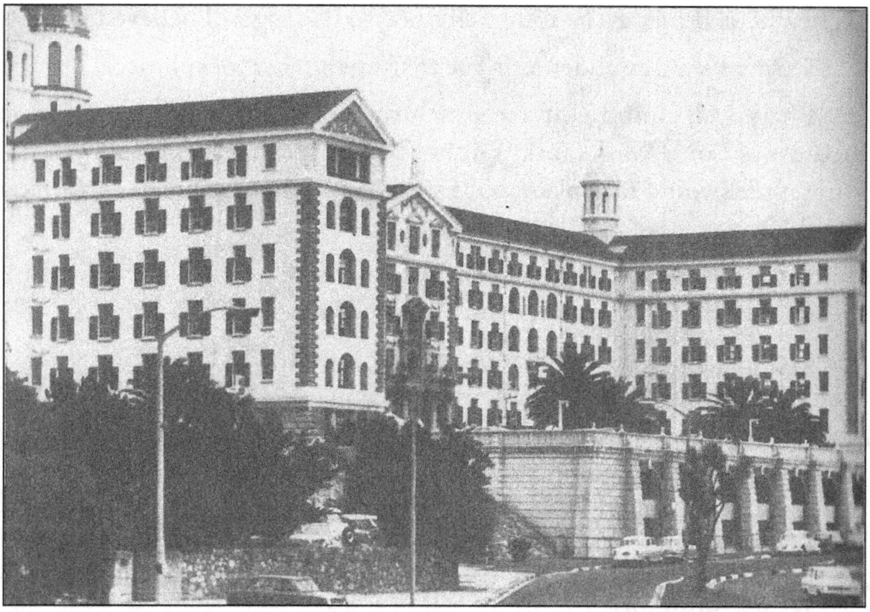

Groote Schuur Hospital, Cape Town—where it all happened.

could help me to go up again as quickly as possible, before I lose my nerve?"

"The sooner the better, Professor Barnard," Phil quickly replied. "I only hope it is a success. As much as I want it to be for my own sake, I want it particularly to be successful for your sake for all that you have done."

"Thank you, Dr. Blaiberg."

I could see Professor Barnard was moved by my husband's spontaneous acceptance of the operation.

As I watched this, I felt I was watching world history in the making. Here was a great drama being played out on the world stage taking place before me and I was one of the few privileged to be in the audience.

"I only ask one thing of you Dr. Blaiberg," Professor Barnard said: "*Moenie skrik nie.* Don't get a fright when you hear I'm going to America tomorrow. I will be back within a few days. I promise you as soon as I get back and we find a donor I will perform the operation. Everything is going to be alright."

Something happened to me that morning during that conversation with Professor Barnard. Before I had been a doubter. Now I was a believer.

When he said that everything was going to be alright, I believed him.

He instilled a confidence in me that was almost inexplicable.

I had been almost convinced that the operation would be called off because of Louis Washkansky's death. Now, a few minutes later, I was not only sure it would take place, but I was ready to believe once more that it would be a success.

Once more I felt on top of the world, although I was sorry for Mrs. Washkansky. I knew how she must have been feeling.

Oh how pleased I was that Phil was going to be given a chance to take hold of a new life, to live and to breathe again like a healthy man. I entered the hospital that day without hope and with little more than a spattering of faith. Now I had both—and they had been given to me by a slim, sad man who had come close to losing his faith.

I held Phil's hand. The thrill of reassurance pulsated through us.

He must not die.

9

Professor Barnard had said: "*Moenie skrik nie*—Don't get a fright." I did not let his visit to America frighten me—at first. But the longer he stayed away, the more my concern increased.

He was away for four days, then five days, then six days. Each seemed like a year.

Phil could hardly breathe now. As I watched him slip ever downwards, I thought his life could be measured in hours.

Daily I prayed over and over again: "Please let him live to have the operation."

A single strand linked Phil with life. That thin strand twined 6,000 miles across the world, where Professor Barnard was addressing millions on television, holding discussions with doctors and defending his actions in performing the first heart transplant.

Could it be that he did not know how ill Phil was? Perhaps he had forgotten Phil's condition in the excitement of world acclaim. He might even think that Phil had a long time to live and could wait patiently for the operation.

"*Moenie skrik nie*" could console me no longer. Desperation seized hold of me as the days dragged on and Phil slowly started losing his hold of that thin strand. Suddenly it could be all over. Then that would be that.

No chance then to call out hysterically to Professor Barnard. The time could only be now. The future lay shrouded in fog. No man had a light strong enough to penetrate it.

I suppose desperation seizes hold of one's mind and turns it giddy so you do things you would normally not do. I know if I had sat down and thought rationally I might not have acted as I did. But I could not think rationally.

I asked a television company to contact Professor Barnard in the United States. I wanted him to know how dangerously ill Phil was. I knew he would want to know. He was our only hope.

I telephoned Professor Schrire.

"Is my husband going to last out?" I said. "I just don't know any longer, so I have asked one of the television companies to send a cable to Professor Barnard. Have I done a terrible thing?"

"If you feel you are telling the truth that is all that matters in this world."

Professor Barnard received the cable. Immediately he did he got in touch with Professor Schrire and asked him whether it was true.

"Yes," Professor Schrire told him. "We are feeding him intravenously to try to keep him going, but it will not be for long."

Nobody in the hospital knew when Professor Barnard would return.

"It might be tomorrow," they said. But so often tomorrow came and went without Professor Barnard.

Every day I heard rumours that he would be returning.

I listened anxiously to the radio and I read the newspapers, trying to find a definite statement to which I could cling, a date to which I could look forward—a goal at which Phil could aim.

Then at last came news that Professor Barnard would return on January 1. Now I had another worry. Once Professor Barnard returned, would they be able to find a donor?

Phil might have to wait many days more until that happened. Would he live that long?

The tense wait sapped my strength and I wondered for how long I would be able to take it without cracking.

On December 28, the hospital staff prepared Phil for the operation. They moved him into a special ward and shaved him from head to toe. Phil was such a hairy man that this took them a full 24 hours, working in shifts.

He laughed at their efforts, saying the way in which they shaved him was the only inefficient part about the whole operation.

He was thrilled, though, because now he could for the first time see more material progress being made towards his having the operation.

"Ah, it is coming nearer," he told me.

But as he waited he became increasingly impatient.

"I don't think the professor is ever coming back" or "I don't think

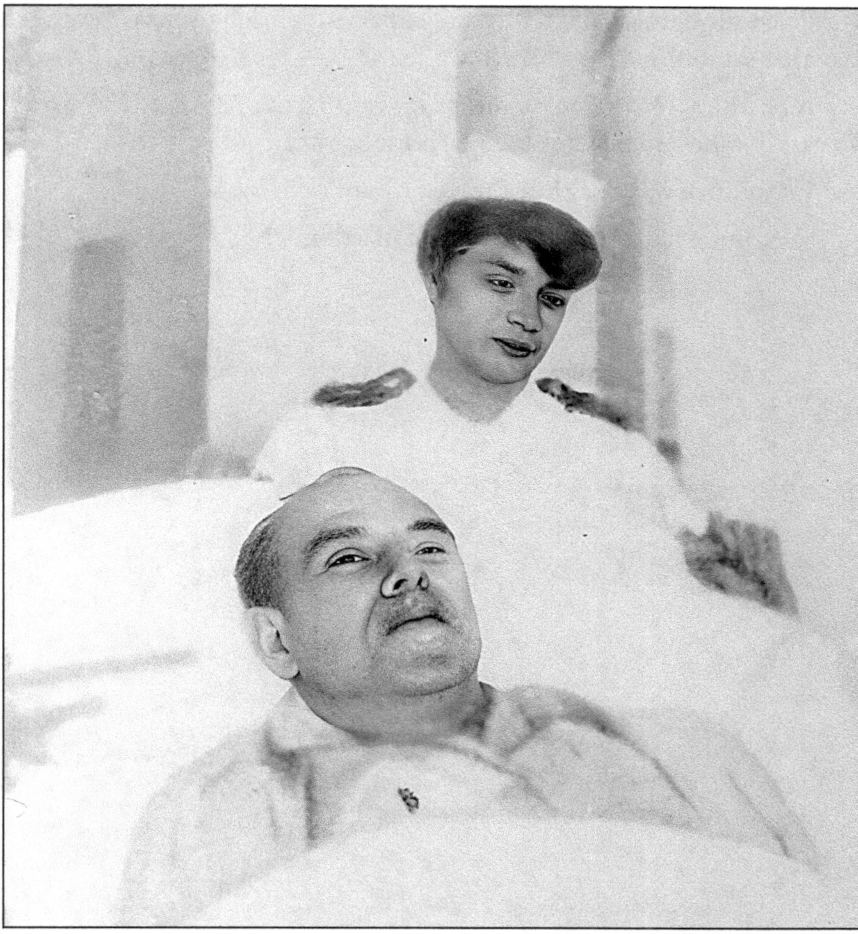

Phil taken to be prepared for surgery

they'll ever find a donor."

Phil was really low at this time. They pumped him with medicines just to keep him alive.

His body was thin and emaciated. Far from being the rosy, cheerful, plump "Father Christmas" that the world later got to know, Phil was then pale, sickly and flat-bellied. It seemed to me he was fading away.

A shudder went through me as I watched the skeleton-like figure struggling to speak, struggling to breathe, struggling to eat, struggling just to live.

Professor Barnard did return on January 1. A bright, sunny New Year's day that symbolised for Phil a new life.

A beardless Old Father Time, he lay gasping the last air of 1967, ready to cast it aside and become the newborn baby of 1968.

"Isn't it marvellous, Phil? Professor Barnard is back."

"Yes, but when are they going to find a donor?"

10

It was New Year's Day, 1968, a public holiday in South Africa and midsummer. Everyone in Cape Town was on vacation. The beaches were packed with holiday makers tanning themselves in the hot sunshine, splashing happily in the cool waves.

New Year's Day and the following day, also a public holiday for most workers in the Cape, belong traditionally to the Coloured folk. Clad in bright coloured raiment, merrily strumming their guitars and singing their tuneful folksongs interspersed with the latest hits, they swing through the city streets for their annual Minstrel Carnival. Large crowds gather to watch and cheer their capers.

For Clive and Dorothy Haupt the New Year Day's treat was to be a trip to Glencairn beach with friends and members of their family. They packed a large picnic basket and set out early to laze in the sun, play on the sands, and swim in the sea.

Clive Haupt had been born on 16 October 1943, one of 11 children of a poor family who lived in a small two-bedroomed cottage in Q Town, Athlone, a large township that forms a suburb of Cape Town.

To the casual observer, the small barefooted lad playing in the Athlone streets was no different from thousands like him.

But to his mother, Mrs Muriel Haupt, he was. From an early age he showed qualities her other children did not. She brought them up well and all were obedient. But Clive, she felt, was a cut above them. He was "specially good".

Certainly he would rough and tumble with the boys. And he was not scared to stand up to someone who wanted to start a fight. But he was considerate where others were thoughtless, mannerly where others were careless. He was peace-loving where others were quarrelsome. These qualities endeared him to everyone. He never sought to push himself. He was not a leader and kept quietly to himself.

When he reached Standard Six he left the North Primary School, Athlone. He had the ability to study further, but it was difficult for his mother, then a widow, to rear her large family.

She needed every penny to ward off starvation. So Clive went out to look for work.

He was 16 when he started his first job at a factory that manufactured breakfast foods. He worked there for three years and after that at a nylon and spinning factory, where he was a machinist.

He had few girl friends. Then he met Dorothy Snyders, a girl of his own age. She was also shy and retiring, and their tastes and interests were alike. They would go to the cinema or spend the evenings at home playing cards.

They had been courting about a year before they became engaged. The big day was 13 August 1966, Dorothy's birthday.

A year later they married in St Luke's Anglican Church. Clive moved from his own home to Dorothy's large house in Portland Street, Salt River, opposite the church.

On holidays friends would call for Clive and Dorothy, who could not afford a car, and take them for drives into the country or to the beach. That was how they came to be at Glencairn that New Year's Day, 1968.

The hours on the beach passed pleasantly. At noon someone started to throw a ball about. Clive joined in with zest.

Laughingly, he dived at his wife's legs. Next moment he lay motionless. "He must have gone to sleep," an onlooker joked. Others said he was fooling. Clive liked a practical joke.

But his wife quickly sensed that something was wrong. She turned him over. He was unconscious. His tongue and mouth were swollen and he frothed at the mouth.

He was hurried by car to the nearest hospital at False Bay.

Doctors summoned an ambulance to take him to the larger Victoria Hospital, in the suburb of Wynberg. His breathing was weak when he reached there at 3.30 p.m.—three and a half hours after his collapse on the beach.

Dr. Basil Sacks, an intern, who examined him, was impressed with his apparent physical fitness and youth. Diagnosing a massive cerebral hemorrhage, he observed that the man's breathing was becoming progressively worse. Ten minutes later it stopped. This sign of respiratory failure indicated irreversible brain damage and death seemed imminent.

As a last resort, Dr. Sacks placed a tube down the man's throat and breathed for him. He was assisted by Dr. J. Filmer, who was also on duty. What impressed the doctors was the manner in which the heart began to beat with the application of oxygen. They expected it to continue, however, for only a brief period under artificial respiration. Once his breathing ceased nothing could be done to save him. But, they reasoned, his heart must be extremely strong for it to have reacted in the way it did.

Dr. Sacks telephoned Dr. Coert Venter, senior registrar of Ward C-2 at Groote Schuur Hospital. "I might have a heart donor for you," he said and described Haupt's condition. He knew a second transplant was imminent and that a donor was being sought.

Five minutes later Dr. Venter was on the telephone. He urged the doctors to do their utmost to keep the patient alive and bring him to Groote Schuur Hospital with all speed. Dr. Sacks accompanied Haupt in the ambulance giving him artificial respiration on the way by ambu bag—used to provide positive pressure ventilation to patients who are not breathing or not breathing properly. With him was a blood sample Dr. Venter had asked him to take before inserting an intravenous drip. This blood was to be used for cross-matching purposes to determine whether it was compatible with that of Phil.

The team had gathered in readiness at the hospital when the ambulance arrived shortly after 5 p.m., and the battle for Clive Haupt's life continued. Dorothy Haupt, her mother, and Muriel Haupt, Clive's mother, sat in a room waiting in anguish for news.

At 7 p.m. it came. Dr. Venter told Dorothy her husband's condition was critical.

The doctors were still fighting to save him, but there was little they could do. An artery had burst in his brain.

It was Dr. Venter's lot to ask her whether she would consent to her husband's heart being used in a transplant operation. Transplant? Her husband dying when only a few short hours before he had been happily picnicking on the beach?

It seemed unreal.

At first the words did not come. She was overwhelmed. Then she sobbed, "If you can save someone else's life in that way, you may take my husband's heart."

She walked over and spoke to Clive's mother. Would she likewise agree to the removal of her son's heart to save a dying man? Her reply, too, was yes.

Tests continued. Doctors, led by Dr. Botha, the team's immunologist, checked their early diagnosis that Clive Haupt's heart would be suitable for transplantation.

A cardiac monitor noted its every beat. Matching tests involving factors for tissue-typing were started.

At 9 p.m. it was decided to re-assess the prognosis later. Clive would die if artificial breathing were stopped.

That in itself was a form of treatment. It would be continued until there was no hope at all of life.

It was an agonizing night for the Haupt family and a tense and anxious one for the transplant team who stood by for a call that might come at any moment.

11

For some reason, I went to the hospital that evening of January 1 earlier than I usually did. The reason for my doing that has become a blank in my mind. It was almost as though I had been led there.

As I sat with Phil, I saw a hub of activity outside the ward. I wondered what was happening. I was soon to find out.

A doctor called me to speak to him in the office. What could it be? Could it be that at last something was about to happen?

"This is it," the doctor whispered, answering my unasked question. "We have found a donor and we think we can start the operation by 11 o'clock tonight."

He was like an excited schoolboy.

A chance—at last.

"Shall I go and tell Phil?"

"No, don't do anything until later, otherwise he will start getting impatient if the operation does not start immediately."

I went back to Phil's room. At that stage I was already wearing a hospital mask to prevent the spread of infection. It was a handy aid to cover my expressions, too.

Phil spoke first.

"I am furious with the doctors. You know what they have done? They have taken away my water."

A glass of water had become precious to Phil. He had always consumed a lot of water before being hospitalised. When the amount of water he could drink was rationed at the hospital he put up a fight.

The tablets made him even thirstier. He was allowed only a specified number of glasses of water a day. These he would divide up into quarters or thirds and then allow himself rations.

Each time I visited him he would proudly tell me how he had improved on his rations.

This night he had succeeded in keeping a half glass of water over for the evening instead of the third he usually had left. He was particularly proud of this.

Then they had taken even that away from him. And he had been looking forward to it so much.

"Everything's cleared away. I don't know how they expect me to sleep tonight. No sleeping tablets, no sedatives, no water. Any moment I'll get out of this bed and walk home."

Underneath the mask I smiled because I knew he could just as much walk home as he could fly to the moon.

"I'll see what I can do," I mumbled. Outside I found Dr. Bosman.

That was the first time I met the doctor who was to become such a personal friend that we always spoke about him as "Bossie".

"I'm afraid you will have to do something because he does not understand why you have taken away everything."

Bossie came back into the room with me. I was then to have my first introduction to the exciting way Bossie could do things.

"Phil," he said. "You know, tonight's the night."

I watched my husband's face. It was as though you had just given him the present he had been asking for all year.

"You rogues," he said. "At last you are going to do something for me. I thought this time would never come."

He looked at me. "Promise me you will not leave me until the operation."

Leaving was furthest from my mind for I was as excited and mixed up as he was.

I promised I would stay.

Dr. Bosman went out of the room, but I followed him a moment later.

"He is so excited there is no sign of his sleeping. I am afraid you will have to give him a sedative," I said.

He agreed with me. Within about a quarter-of-an-hour Phil was asleep.

At 8 o'clock that night the doctors were excitedly coming and going from the vicinity of Phil's ward. Some moved equipment or instruments. Others were talking. All were excited.

I had brought nothing with me and I was feeling cold. I told a doctor that I would be going home quickly to fetch my coat.

I asked whether someone could watch Phil and if he awoke tell him that I would be back soon.

The doctor laughed. "He will sleep right through until the morning."

But I was terrified that Phil would awaken without me and ask for me. I went home as quickly as I could and fetched my coat, ready for the night's vigil at Phil's bedside.

It is not easy to sit in a chair for a long time at night when you are not accustomed to it.

Every hour or half-hour I would take a break, go into the passage to light a cigarette or take a breath of air.

Always I remained close to the door with an eye on Phil.

During those quiet hours I had time to think about what was happening around me.

For the first time the obvious struck me: They must have found a donor.

But who is he?

Where is he?

Where is his family?

At one stage I wanted to ask one of the doctors the answers to these questions, but then I thought again. I didn't really want to know. I didn't want to become involved with someone else's sorrow. The less I knew about it the better.

At one time when I came out into the passage, however, I saw a crowd of people a few doors away, down the passage. They looked sad.

From a ward near where they stood I could hear the monotonous "beep-beep" of a machine registering someone's heart beat. Was it registering the heart beat my husband was soon to have?

By that time the doctors had left. I did not think I should ask the nurses.

Eventually I decided I would not ask anybody. Nobody said anything. I sensed they were happy that I did not question them. It could have been a difficult situation had I met the family of the donor that evening.

About 10 o'clock my brother, Abe, and my brothers-in-law, Ben and Harry, arrived.

They told me they had to push their way through a barrage of television and newspapermen outside. They were shocked to think that they could not even give us some privacy at a time like that.

Throughout the night the hospital was surrounded by TV reporters and print journalists. How they got wind of the impending operation only they know.

I have learned, from experience, however, you can't keep a story from men with a nose for news. They refuse to accept vague statements.

Nurses had to order them from the passage where Phil's and the donor's wards were located. They were threatened with the police.

Still they prowled about. Telephone calls were booked to London and New York to catch the latest editions of newspapers.

For me, though, it was no story, no matter what impact it made on the world. It was my husband's life. The hours had never passed so slowly. Eleven o'clock came and went. Then it was midnight. Still there was no word to relieve my suspense.

Dr. Marius Barnard, Christiaan's brother and also a heart surgeon, came to me later that evening and said, "From now on there is going to be no such thing as privacy for you. I think you will have to live somewhere anonymously, because they will kill you with all this publicity."

I was not worried about that at that stage. There were more immediate concerns. Just let the operation pass, I thought, then we will turn our attention to that problem.

I still had not seen Professor Barnard that evening, but doctors regularly made appearances.

You could sense the excitement throbbing through them all. A nurse answering the telephone, a reporter being told firmly that the passage was barred to the public. Nothing more.

Two o'clock and my sixth cup of coffee. Now everything was quiet, quite different, I would imagine, from a normal night at the hospital.

A doctor whom I did not know came to me shortly after 2 a.m.

"Mrs. Blaiberg, you will have to go home," he said. "You just cannot go on like this. All the doctors have gone home because it looks as though it will not take place until tomorrow morning."

"No, I can't do that."

"Do me a favour and go and get some sleep while you can. You will need your energy later today."

"No, I promised Phil I would stay at his bedside until the operation. What if he should wake up and call me? I will never forgive myself if I am not here."

"Look, Mrs. Blaiberg, he is so drugged. He will not call you."

It took more persuasion, but finally I agreed.

"Let me give you a lift home," he offered.

It was about 2.45 a.m. when I got home, exhausted.

Before I went to sleep, I thought, I must write to Jill and tell her that the operation was now going to take place.

I sat writing to her until 5.30 a.m. I don't know what I wrote, but I guess I must have explained everything to her, telling her not to worry, I would contact her and again try to telephone her once it was over.

I crawled exhausted into bed, filled with worry, misery—and coffee.

It was 9.30 a.m. when the telephone awoke me.

"Come immediately."

My sister, who had come down from Port Elizabeth to be with me, drove me to the hospital.

My big concern then was that he might have woken up to find me not there. Had I let him down?

When we got into the hospital they were putting Phil on the trolley. He was awake. So I had let him down.

The doctors assured me, however, that he had just woken up. In any event, I think he was so mixed up and he was so excited that he did not realise I had not been there.

Our parting must have been one of the coldest two lovers have ever had. The reason: A nurse was standing right next to us, which made it embarrassing for either of us to show much emotion.

He waved to me. "Goodbye".

I smiled at him.

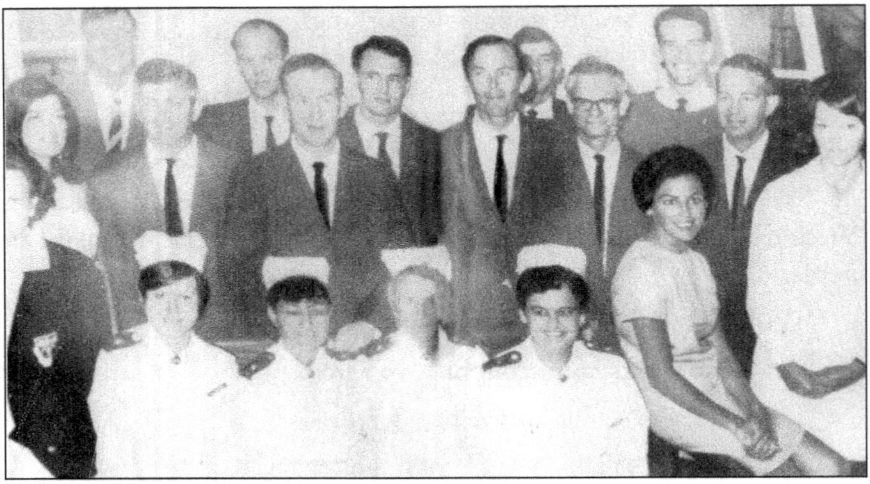

The heart team: Doctors, anesthesiologists, nurses. The success of the undertaking was due, in large measure, to the expertise and dedication of the people who worked on it: Researchers, physicians, technicians, and young women fresh out of nursing school. Each of these individuals became a precise cog within the great "machine" directed by Dr. Christiaan Barnard (centre).

"Aren't you going to kiss him goodbye, Mrs. Blaiberg?" asked the nurse.

I leaned down and kissed him. "Goodbye and lots of luck."

That should have been a dramatic farewell. There was, after all, the chance that we might never have seen one another again.

Yet we both acted as though Phil was on his way to work. I was trying to be as matter-of-fact about the whole thing as I could, as though it was nothing.

Phil was wheeled down the passage on the trolley, waving to the nurses, wildly excited.

The nurse who had been with us when we parted turned to me. "Mrs. Blaiberg, you said goodbye so ordinarily."

A shock wave tore through my mind. What had I done?

I was the one who had been pushing the idea of a transplant all the time.

Perhaps he would live only another two or three weeks and therefore I might have sent him to a certain death.

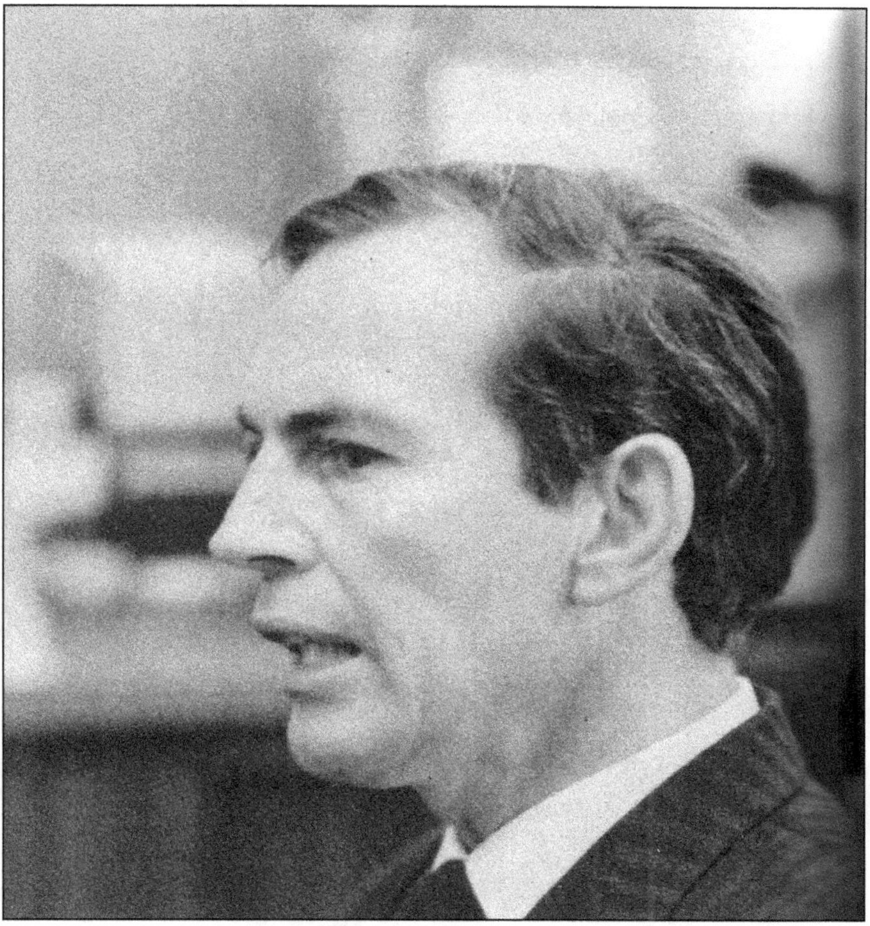

Barnard discusses the transplant.

How could I be sure that the operation would be a success?

A feeling of guilt pervaded me. I had forced my husband to take a step that might mean his end?

Tiredness, dismay, frustration burst together in a frenzy. I cried great tears of unhappiness in what should have been a time of joy.

I wept and I wept.

For once I allowed myself a measure of self-pity. Before I had left the flat I had telephoned the doctor, and asked him to prescribe a strong sleeping tablet for me.

There was one thing I was certain of and that was that I was determined not to live through that operation in a wakeful state.

I went home, took the tablet and got straight into bed.

I fell into a deep sleep. Now it was up to the doctors.

12

It was 3.30 that afternoon, January 2, when I awoke with a start. A crowd of people stood around me and at first I was not quite sure where I was.

"Congratulations." they shouted.

Congratulations? Oh yes, Phil.

"What happened?" I asked eagerly. Now I was properly awake and anxious to know the outcome.

"We have just heard on the radio that the operation was a complete success," they said. "The heart started beating of its own accord without an electric shock."

I looked around at their delighted faces, but I found it difficult to raise their sort of enthusiasm.

Are you people mad? What are you excited about? What are you celebrating?

"The long road ahead is only starting now." It hit me forcibly then that the operation was only the technical beginning. Had Louis Washkansky not died after 18 days? What were these people getting so excited about? I became so irritable that I thought the best thing was to get out of the room because they could not feel about it as I did.

How can other people think for you when the person is really your very own?

The long uphill struggle lay ahead. What did I think of at that moment when I knew Phil's life had been spared, that my prayers had been answered, that the barest flicker of hope had been rekindled?

At first I was too stunned to grasp the immensity and wonder of it. Then, gradually, the prospect and possibility of a future life together with Phil spread out before me. Can any of you imagine what a feeling of relief and gladness that was for a woman who had accepted, for nine months, that she would have to live the rest of her life without her loved one?

My friends telephoned and crowded our apartment to celebrate. The champagne corks popped. They were delirious with joy and excitement and toasted me and Phil. They drank to his good health and many more years of life. I thanked them; but I told them it was not yet time for celebration, only thankfulness. I realised only too well, although I don't think they did understand at the time, the hazards that lay ahead.

I recalled the excitement after the operation on Louis Washkansky and how tragically it ended. I was determined to remain level-headed, not to give way to over-optimism, to wait and see how things developed during the next few weeks.

I did not know at that time that a comparatively easy passage lay before us. Every day I feared, or expected, some complication or setback. When I spoke to the doctors at the hospital they sounded elated and assured me all was well.

I breathed a prayer of relief but I said to myself, "Eileen, just wait another few days before you get delirious about it all."

And that is just what I did. I knew that no one, not even the doctors, could predict the course of events in the next few days and weeks and what the effects of the immunosuppressive drugs would be.

Anything could go wrong at any time. No one could give me any guarantees.

Each day I awoke with the thought, "What is today going to bring?"

13

For the first18 days of the way Phil would set his steps in the footsteps of Louis Washkansky. Those were the number of days that Washkansky had been alive. But from there on the ground was untrodden, smooth like a beach after the high tide has washed over it. I hoped, but dared not hope too strongly, that Phil would be able to make the first imprints on that unchartered way.

There was little basis for me, not being a doctor, to regard Phil's transplant as more successful than that of Washkansky. Why, therefore, should he have so much more life ahead of him?

After the operation Phil was moved into the transplant unit, a sterile suite in the outpatients' ward of the hospital. I telephoned the hospital about five times a day. In fact, I often wondered at their patience in answering my regular calls so sympathetically. I would just say: "It's Mrs. Blaiberg" and they would put me through to the transplant unit.

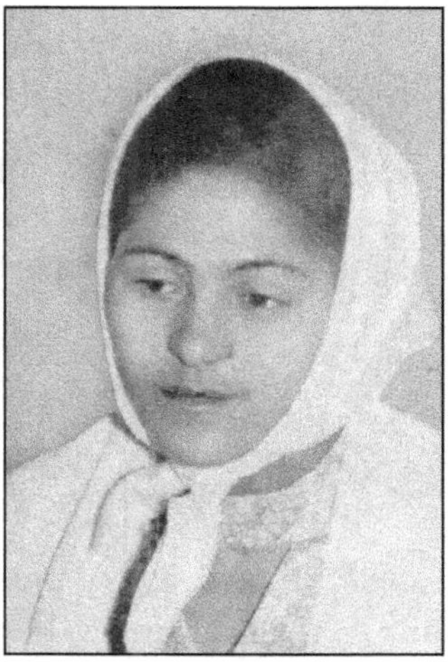

Dorothy Haupt—Her husband's heart continued to beat in Phil's chest.

The report was always encouraging: "He is doing marvellously." I never worried to ask them when I would be able to go to the hospital and see Phil. I thought after the experience of the previous transplant they would want to be ultra careful in not passing on any infection to him. As far as I was concerned his health was more important than not being able to see him.

The saddest part of that time was when I attended Clive Haupt's funeral. That was one of the greatest ordeals I had to face during the whole 19 months following the transplant. I went to the funeral that day with fear pounding in my heart. How was I going to be received by the Coloured people? Here I was going to the funeral and my husband was alive with the heart of the man they were burying.

Would they resent me, turn a cold shoulder on me? What was it going to be like?

When I arrived there my fear grew greater. It was the first time I had ever had to face a crowd like that. Onlookers filled the road outside the church; they sat on rooftops and they lined the streets for blocks around—15,000 of them.

But what surprised me was the warmth with which I was received that day. From the church service, right to the cemetery. Thousands of people tried to get near to me to touch my hand and wish my husband well. What a difference it was from what I had imagined. They really made me feel as though they genuinely were with me and wanted Phil to live.

In fact, during the whole 19 months of Phil's post-operative life that was the kind of reception we got from the Coloured community wherever we went. Always they would inquire about "the doctor", meaning Phil. It became almost a love they had for him. I think it was because he was so natural with them when they asked him for his autograph, for example. He was particularly pleasant toward the Coloured people after his transplant because he felt he owed them something. They could feel this warmth flowing from him and this developed into a bond of affection.

The transplant team suggested that I might be able to visit Phil on the fifth day after the transplant. I waited excitedly for that day.

Finally it came and I went to the hospital. The transplant unit had been created in premises formerly occupied by the ear, nose and throat section of the out-patients' department. It was at the end of a long passage.

When I reached the start of the passage, I was surprised to find a policeman guarding it.

"Who are you?" he asked. I felt as though I was entering a military encampment.

With that, one of the doctors came from somewhere and introduced me to the policeman. He told him that whenever I came in the future I should immediately be admitted. The doctor also called the policeman from the other end of the passage and introduced him to me as well.

By then I almost felt I was walking on holy ground. When I reached the unit, I was introduced to the ritual that preceded entry into the "holy of holies" in which Phil was being cared for. First I put on boots, then I had to walk into some disinfectant. From there I went into another room where my mask and hood were put on. In a third room, the nurse took out a packet in which there was a gown. Barely touching the sterilised gown with her gloves, the sister put the gown on me. After it had been fastened up the back, I had to wash my hands. Over my hands, I wore rubber gloves.

After this elaborate ritual, I looked forward to walking into my husband's room where we would meet for the first time since the operation. I was already shaking from excitement. But the fear of infection was so great that, in spite of taking all these precautions, I was not allowed to enter his room. Instead, I had to speak to him through a glass partition from a passage outside his room.

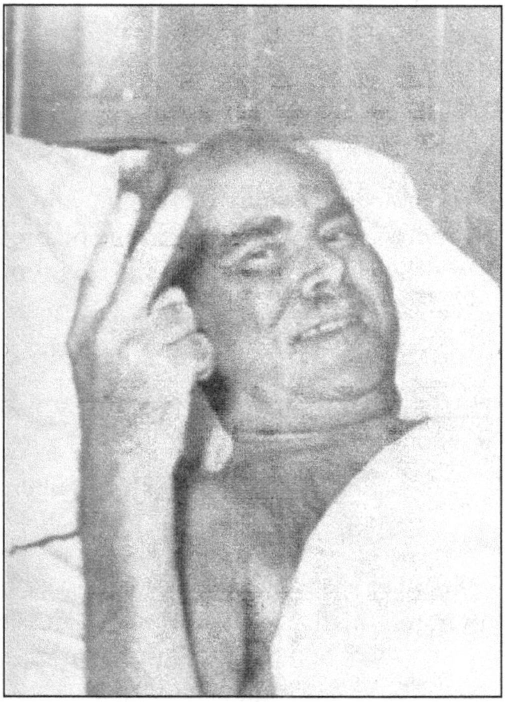

Phil gives the V-sign for victory after the transplant.

That is how I had to speak to him for two-and-a-half months.

On the first visit I was too overcome to say much. His complexion was radically different from the last time I had seen him. His eyes were blue with the blueness that had made my heart skip a beat in those early Oudtshoorn days where we grew up. I felt I was falling in love with him all over again. He looked about 10 years younger—and I felt a rejuvenation myself.

"From now on life is going to be too wonderful," he said.

I found it a slight strain talking loudly through the glass partition. Later they moved his bed forward, closer to the partition. This was followed by the luxury of an intercom. At first it was fun, but we discontinued it because I did not feel natural turning it on and off to speak to each other.

As I came out of the transplant unit that day, one of the registrars asked, "Is Jill coming back to Cape Town?"

"Well, my husband didn't want her to come under any circumstances, whether he made the operation or not," I replied.

"You know, I think he needs just that little extra stimulus," the registrar said. "Then he will be really well. You can go and ask him if he would like her to come."

The next day I visited Phil. I asked him. His eyes lit up. "Let her come, even if it is for a few days, just let me see her again," he said.

I cabled Jill, asking her to come home. She received quite a shock at receiving it, for only a short time before I had written and told her that under no circumstances was she to return home. But Phil was well now.

She hardly knew what to pack—her brush, books that she needed to study, only one change of clothing. She left that same night in a whirl.

In the meantime I visited Phil every morning. Each day when I would walk out of the building a group of reporters stood outside, eager for news.

"What did he say today, Mrs. Blaiberg?"

"He is fine, never felt better."

And so it went every day. I did not know quite what to say. Phil locked up in the small transplant unit could scarcely produce a crop of exciting news breaks. He simply continued to progress each day.

What more could I tell the press?

I used to tell him a bit of news of the outside world, but all he could report to me were things like: The doctors are good, the nurses are fabulous, the food is appetising. Those facts were not calculated to make world-shattering news.

One day when I went to visit him I asked him: "Say something different today, please darling."

He looked at me as if I had had too much sun. "What are you talking about? What do you mean: Say something different?"

"These newspapermen are on at me all the time. If they are not waiting downstairs, they phone the minute I get home."

"Why is it so important what I say? What do they want me to do?"

Phil could not yet grasp what an impact his operation had made on

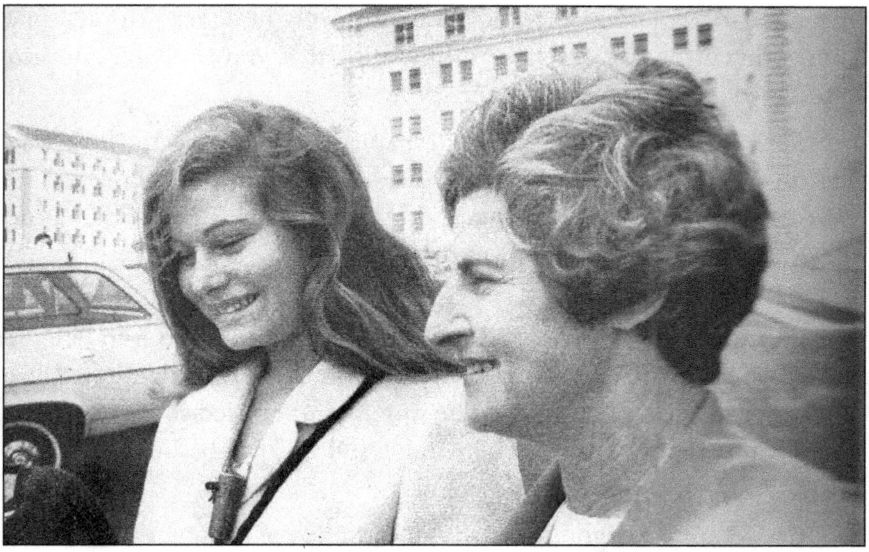

Jill and Eileen Blaiberg outside Groote Schuur Hospital

the world. True, he had heard about Washkansky's operation, but somehow when it happens to you it is different. He did not expect the world to get as excited as it did. When I told him about the newspapermen, it did not register to him that the world could be so interested. He thought that once the first transplant was over his would be taken for granted.

In an effort to get him to understand what was going on, I would tell him about the piles of telegrams that were arriving and the flood of letters in the mail daily.

"I don't know," he said. "This is a crazy world. Whatever are they so interested for? I'm fine. I've just got a new pump and that is all there is to it."

But, crazy or not, the longer he lived the more the world got excited about it and the more letters arrived for him.

Jill arrived about the eighth day after the operation took place, and that made a little more news again. And it shocked Jill, too. She thought she was getting away from the newsmen in Israel. But when she arrived at the airport in Cape Town a crowd of hungry newsmen were awaiting her.

I was at the airport to meet her. We were both ushered into the V.I.P. room where we were subject to questioning, photographing and filming.

This was a new world for us. It is all very well being royalty or a politician or someone like that, but to be suddenly flung into the centre of the world's attention because of something that you really had nothing directly to do with yourself is unnerving.

When Phil saw Jill, he cried unashamedly. Then it hit me how weak he still was. The more Phil cried, the more Jill cried. I saw how wet her mask had become from her tears and I told her to change it. She was not allowed to stay there with a wet mask on because every little germ was being carefully watched.

That was the man who said it did not matter much to him whether Jill returned. Now I knew how much it meant to him and that it had been a sacrifice to say that. Of course he cared, but he cared so much that he did not want her to interrupt her studies in Israel just because he was undergoing an operation.

The doctor was right. It did a lot for Phil to see Jill again at that stage.

Jill stayed for eight days. During that time she came with me to the hospital every day to see Phil. Her brief stay provided a diversion for the press, but soon it was back to the same question: "Didn't he say something different today?"

Again I asked him whether he could not think of something new to say.

"Well, you just tell the reporters this: Before I had my heart attack, I climbed Lion's Head overlooking Cape Town. After I come out of here I am going to climb the highest peak. That is how fit I feel."

Then the reporters wanted details of his menus and his appetite. I told them. Next day the products of the Groote Schuur Hospital kitchens, as delivered to Phil in his suite, were quoted throughout the continents.

Once I mentioned that Phil enjoyed a hearty breakfast. This, too, became world news. A woman in Australia assumed that his "hearty breakfast" included a plentiful helping of bacon and eggs, toast and marmalade, tea or coffee. She wrote warning him against the perils of the breakfast tray and urged him, above all, to avoid bacon. Phil never ate it.

All the time I was being photographed wherever I went, entering and leaving the hospital, shopping, lunching, and dining, I became heartily sick of my face staring at me from the newspapers. But the photographers had their instructions and duties. I was trailed, "shot", and, once more, I was in the papers. Phil was highly amused. I wasn't.

"Now you know what kings and queens have to put up with," he grinned. "They can have it," I said with feeling. "And it's all my fault," Phil apologized.

The world, I found, continued to be publicity and news crazy. A fierce and ever-increasing competition developed among newspapers, magazines, radio, and television for a "beat" on the Blaiberg Story. Even my own daily doings, many trivial, were page-one news.

Well, I decided, if that was the way it had to be, there was nothing for me but to resign myself to it.

My attempt to avoid the deluge before Phil's operation had landed me in a spot of bother with some newspapers. They believed I was withholding news from them because of some contract I had made, whereas the truth was simply that I desperately wanted to avoid the operation being turned into some sort of circus stunt.

I found life much easier when I let the press have what they wanted when they wanted it. I couldn't argue with them and carry my worries and burdens at the same time. Though there were exceptions, I must add that reporters and television teams were polite, helpful and considerate. If you are frank with them, explain your difficulties and problems, they will respect your confidences. They had a job to do and, as Phil said, we should help them all we could.

I learned to be absolutely accurate in every word I said. If I happened to make a remark that seemed to be incorrect, I knew there would be thousands who would certainly let me know. For months letters would arrive demanding an explanation as to why I said this or that.

It did not hit home to Phil at that time how much the world was interested in him. He was too engrossed in his little world. At that stage he was not even listening to the radio, let alone reading newspapers. Indeed, it was to be two months before he started listening to the radio.

Then the eighteenth day—the day on which Louis Washkansky had died—came closer. Slowly it loomed larger as it got nearer, assuming symbolic significance. I have always been almost stupidly superstitious.

Just after Jill left—and just as the eighteenth day was starting to loom on the horizon—Phil developed a sore throat. The doctors told me they did not think it was anything to worry about, but they were not sure what it was.

Though Phil made light of his sore throat it was, while it lasted, a nightmare to me and the entire transplant unit. Our nerves were on edge. I telephoned the doctors constantly, every hour, to inquire about him. I could not sleep at night thinking of the possible causes and the grim implications. At the back of our minds, I suppose, was the fear of an infection that might have fatal consequences.

I can talk about it calmly now, but I will never forget my anxiety and downright pessimism then. Sometimes I thought it the beginning of the end. Had Phil come so far, undergone a successful transplant operation, only to... I tried to stop my thoughts at that point. After my restless nights, however, there was Phil waiting for me, his usual, bright self, wearing his jolly smile.

"How is your throat?"

"It's all right." he said. "It's nothing. There's nothing to worry about. Just a little irritation. It'll go away. You'll see."

I played along with him. I pretended I also believed it was not serious. I would not allow him, for a moment, to guess my thoughts. I believe he thought he had convinced me that there was "nothing to it", nothing, really, to concern myself about.

But the doctors could not pretend. They suffered as I did. Some of them, too, had sleepless nights. The slightest abnormality in Phil, a point up in his temperature, an ache or pain he had not known the day before—all were of the greatest concern to them.

They admitted they had nothing to guide them. At that time Phil was the only living man with a transplanted heart. Who knew what problems might suddenly, and unexpectedly, arise in spite of all the drugs and treatment given him? There were always the imponderables and the unpredictables.

Whether the doctors told me or not, I somehow knew, probably by intuition, when things were not going well or as well as they hoped.

Sometimes I drove away from the hospital in a state of nerves and tension, leaving behind a husband who did not seem to have a care in the world, who said good-bye to me with a smile and a jest. But I always sensed when the doctors were worried. Looking back on those days I am forever thankful that our fears were false alarms as Phil said they were.

If only I had been able to show his courage and optimism, how much less I would have suffered.

Up to now, everything had gone so well. Now, as the eighteenth day neared, it held trouble in its right hand. Few would be so brave as to wave the trouble aside for they were all on unchartered ground in which the signs were not erected by doctors who had travelled that way before. The signs were in a foreign tongue no man could read. Could this sore throat be a danger sign?

I telephoned Professor Barnard to seek some assurance. It was something I should never have done. For he was the one who needed reassuring.

"Professor, how is my husband?" I asked.

"He is just not well." That's all.

I realised then that if I ever wanted comfort, Professor Barnard was not the one to whom I should turn. For he became more worried than I was.

"Has he ever had shingles before?" Professor Barnard asked me hastily. "Has he ever had sores on his lips before?" The questions came with the rapidity of gunfire. Has he ever had this before? Has he ever had that before?

He got me so muddled that I could scarcely think what my husband had had before.

"I think he has had sores on his lips before."

"Oh, thank goodness for that. Then it can't be so serious."

I could hear him sigh with relief. Far from getting assistance from him, about dates and just the thought of the eighteenth day, he disturbed me. I still felt worried, so I telephoned one of Professor Barnard's registrars.

"Please, Mrs. Blaiberg, don't be worried. It's not anything serious. Don't let Professor Barnard's manner upset you. He just panics sometimes, like a parent. Both you and he are like two anxious parents fussing over your sick child. It is no good one anxious parent trying to comfort the other anxious parent."

It appeared that, in fact, the sore throat and the sores on his lips were unimportant. Both soon healed.

The eighteenth day dawned. I decided I would not say anything to the doctors or the nurses. I would just hold my breath and hope for the best. I would go up to the hospital as usual and not pay any attention to the fact that this day held significance for me.

I was fearful of what I would find when I got there. I need not have worried.

"Look at him," the nurses said.

"The eighteenth day has come and gone. He is as well as he could be. Isn't it wonderful?"

Their mention of the day and their evident relief made me realise they, too, had been worried about that day.

It was not long before the eighteenth day and all its imagined terrors had safely passed us by. We continued on our journey, looking now for the next milestone, which was the time he would be discharged from the hospital. I looked forward, too, to the time when I would be allowed to go into his room and not talk to him through the glass partition.

I told them I did not want to rush anything. I was happy to sit at the door and talk to him as long as he was doing well.

I realised he was getting better when he became more avid for news each time I got there. I could also tell his progress by what he came to call his "firsts"—the first day he sat up, the first day he got out of bed, the first day he shaved himself. Each little step was like that taken by a baby. And each was reported in the newspapers.

On most of my visits to Groote Schuur Hospital in a car with a special driver placed at my disposal for three months, I thought I noticed an improvement in Phil. Sometimes it was slight, but the doctors confirmed, from their charts and records, that his progress was continual and my spirits rose. I could smile a genuine smile. I knew he could "see" it even behind my surgical mask—and I did not have to force a smile as I had for so many months.

My visits seemed to stimulate him, and as I sat chatting through the intercom and watched the attention given him by the doctors and nurses I was filled with gratitude. They far exceeded the bounds of duty.

Even in the early days when he was so weak he had a quip for me, the doctors, nurses, everyone. He told me with pride how his breathing was improving all the time as a result of his exercises and how his legs were responding to treatment.

"Eileen," he said one day, "you can't believe what it means to be able to breathe again without suffering."

During all the time he spent in his suite, I don't remember a word of complaint from him. I was surprised one day, about two weeks after the operation, when he said, "Oh, how wonderful it is to be without pain."

"What do you mean?" I asked. "You've never complained about pain before."

"Well, naturally, the wound down my chest was a bit uncomfortable, and I found it difficult to turn in my bed.

"But", he added with a smile, "it's gone now."

That was typical of him. He always declared he had no pain or discomfort until it was over so that I would not worry after I left him.

I learned to have more respect for him on those daily visits than in all our years together. I realised what a stoical and uncomplaining husband I had.

The doctors and nurses agreed he was an ideal patient in every way. They were sure his progress was also largely due to his unconcern about his own suffering and his spirit of determination to get well and over every hurdle as he reached it. The most menial member of the staff found him jolly and full of fun and he tried to make the duties of the nurses as pleasant as possible. It was most unusual, they told me, to find this consideration in a patient as ill as Phil.

One day, I remember, during Jill's visit, he said he had a "big surprise" for us.

"I want you to watch very carefully," he said. "I'm going to walk for you. That'll show you!"

It was a pathetic sight as we saw him lean on two nurses and take a few faltering steps with a smile of happiness on his face. Afterwards, I believe, he asked a nurse whether he had put on a good performance.

If he had only known how Jill and I sobbed after we left. We could not control our tears. He had such pride in his "big surprise". It made us feel humble that such a little achievement could have meant so much to him.

A few weeks later, after Jill had returned to Israel, he told me he had fixed a little mirror to the wall and shaved himself without the aid of the nurses. That was another "milestone", as he called it, along the road to recovery. It was such a small thing, but it again gave him such happiness. It showed Progress, he said, with a capital P.

One day Miss Sternweiler, a physical therapist, brought a two-step "staircase" to Phil's suite. He was to try to climb it. That was his Everest. At first it was an exhausting effort and beyond his strength to climb even the first step unaided. Eventually he succeeded.

Phil had to learn to hasten slowly. Once he almost tumbled off the staircase. Fortunately, Miss Sternweiler and a nurse held on to him and prevented a fall. Still he went on trying.

At last came victory. He conquered the second step as well. Now he stood on top of his little world. No mountaineer at the pinnacle of a perilous climb was prouder than he was.

He did physiotherapy regularly. At first they woke him three or four times a night to do his exercises.

He complained about the disturbances that created, so they made him do his exercises more in the daytime and less at night. The aim was to loosen his joints for the days when he would walk about again.

The therapy paid dividends. When he did get out of bed, although he was wobbly, he had little trouble with walking.

It was a day of great excitement when he had his first meal out of bed about seven weeks after the operation. Once again it was relayed to a still-interested world.

Phil never forgot one incident. Professor Barnard walked into his room, masked and dressed in his usual sterile outfit, carrying a transparent plastic box. In it was Phil's old heart in a preservative solution. Outside, behind the glass panel in the passage, was an official photographer similarly garbed, who was to record the occasion.

Professor Barnard sat next to Phil on his bed and examined his former heart with cool professional interest.

He showed him that more than 90 per cent of the muscle had become fibrosed or converted into functionless scarred tissue. When Professor J. G. Thomson (Pathologist to Groote Schuur Hospital and Head of the Department of Pathology, University of Cape Town) saw it he said that, had he not known it was removed from Phil's chest, he would have declared it was from a corpse. How Phil had managed to remain alive until the transplant was a miracle in itself.

Professor Barnard looked up and said quizzically, "Dr. Blaiberg, do you realise that you are the first man, in the history of mankind to be able to sit, as you are now, and look at his own, dead, heart?"

Believe it or not Phil was so interested, perhaps shocked, by the appearance and condition of his heart that he had not given a thought to the historic implications.

"Now that you mention it," he said somewhat abashed, "it had not occurred to me that I have been looking at my heart."

The photographer's bulbs flashed and the occasion was captured for posterity. The heart itself is now a celebrated pathological specimen.

About four weeks after the operation, some of the doctors told Phil and me that he might be allowed to go home in the near future. How thrilled we were! But the weeks dragged by and turned into months and still nothing happened. It was a strain not knowing when the Great Day would arrive. Now I was put off with "maybe next week". Next week came and went. Still Phil remained in his suite.

Besides the uncertainty, which was hard enough to bear, the press now started to nag and calls came not only from South African newspapers but from all over the world for the top-secret date. Some editors were convinced I knew but would not disclose it, that I had a scoop up my sleeve for some favoured publication. It just wasn't true. I knew as little as they did.

As the weeks passed, I realised that my life and the world I had known were changing. I was dined and wined by journalists and V.I.P.s until I think I knew the menus of every restaurant and hotel grill room in Cape Town. It became almost a standing joke that you could, or should, ask Eileen Blaiberg where to get the best meal in town.

In this new world I gained a host of new and good friends, many among the doctors and nurses at Groote Schuur Hospital. I took along cake for our little tea parties when I visited Phil. I made many other worthy friends in those 74 days, and their friendship and kindness to me and to Phil are something we continue to cherish.

What pleased me most was that, as a result of my new status as wife of a celebrity, I was able to help publicize a number of good causes. For example, I took part in a campaign for blood on behalf of the Western Province Blood Transfusion Service, which played a vital role in the operation.

I was bled on a couch alongside the Acting State President, Mr. Tom Naude, another veteran blood donor, and we were photographed together. That was one photograph I welcomed.

I believe the publicity increased the number of donors. The sequel for me, personally, was not particularly pleasant. When I visited Phil later I almost blacked out. I had been overtaxing myself. However, Phil suspected nothing, gave me a figurative pat on the back for my efforts, and I soon recovered.

I had a glimpse, too, of the wonderful world of television which, at that time, we did not have in South Africa. I gave an interview that was shown throughout the world, and along came shoals of mail wishing Phil well. Jill, too, was televised in Israel and I soon had letters about my "beautiful daughter".

It seems strange that though millions of televiewers had seen and heard Phil and me, we had yet to see ourselves as others saw us. We thought that perhaps, one day, before those films passed into the archives we would be able to relive those days in some television studio in the United States or Britain or Japan. Or, perhaps, we would have television in South Africa.

14

Phil was like a recluse from the outside world during those days he spent in the sterile suite. His windows were opaque and so he could not watch the passing show outside. And yet he never grumbled.

Never did he say to me that he was fed-up with the whole business, He was always optimistic about it. "Soon I will be coming home," he would say.

I think those two-and-half months in the hospital seemed longer to me than they did to Phil. He lived in a little world of his own, not realising what was going on outside.

Finally, the doctors said, "Professor Barnard's returning home tomorrow. The day after he returns, we will let Phil go home. There is nothing to make us keep him here any longer."

At last the time had come for us to be close again. He would bring that strength of purpose, that kind nature, that strength of principle back into our home once more. My prayers had been answered; he was alive. But now I wanted him for my own. I wanted to draw on his strength, relax in the knowledge that, simply, he was there and all that meant. Oh, those lucky nurses. To have had him for so long to inspire them, to make them laugh and to make them sing with the joy of life and to make them love life...for Phil loved life with an infectious love.

Professor Barnard called me into his office when he arrived. "I think we might let him go in a few days time."

"What?" It was as though he had said "a few months' time." He did not understand; I wanted Phil now. "But," I said, "The doctors have already told him, and they have told me, that you would let him go home the day after you returned. That is tomorrow."

"All right," Professor Barnard said. "It will be tomorrow. But now we have no time to waste."

He got in touch with Dr. Nel, who had already done some of the spade work in organising the police, warning them to be ready for the crowd expected to watch as Phil went home. He had also done a lot of the other organising that was necessary.

When he received Professor Barnard's call that day he had to set everything in motion immediately so nobody would be caught on the wrong foot. In fact, the security covering Phil's discharge from the hospital was so important that we had a meeting with top hospital executives to arrange things so that it would all go smoothly and Phil would not be molested by eager crowds wanting to get close enough to touch him or simply by crowds that had got out of hand.

Eventually the day came—March 16, 1968. Trembling with excitement, I packed clothes for Phil. He had been in his pajamas up to now. Clearly he could not face the world on his first day out of hospital dressed in his pajamas.

I went to the hospital and dressed as usual in my special boots, sterile gown, mask and hood. A nurse handed me a list of all the medicines Phil was to have, the times they were to be taken, and how they were to be taken. I wondered how I would ever be able to remember all those names. But I did not know, or really care, what she was telling me. I was too excited for that. I noticed that she was also shaking with excitement.

With that Professor Barnard walked in, his famous smile stretched across his face. "Why have you all got these gowns and masks on? Dr. Blaiberg is going out into the germ-infested world. What are you all being stupid about?"

We looked at him and then laughed. Getting dressed in those sterile gowns and masks had become such a habit we had not even stopped to think that that day was different. So we took off our masks and went in to see Phil.

"Goodness, it's good to see your face again," he said. For two months he had seen only my eyes, reading in them my smiles and my frowns.

Then he turned to the nurses. "Gee, you're beautiful. And, gosh, you're a blonde." They, too, had previously been only eyes.

When he put on his trousers, the fun began. Phil had put on so much weight in the hospital that he could not zip them up.What a wonderful excuse it was to laugh. The atmosphere was tense. This was just what we needed to break the tension by laughing out loud.

But the laughing stopped when we looked out of the windows and saw crowds of cameramen, pressmen, TV reporters, and inquisitive spectators crushing one another to get as close as possible to the floor to get a glimpse of Phil as he came out. We looked back at Phil. What were we going to do? Getting a tailor to alter the trousers was out of the question now; yet so was Phil going out in his pajamas. He could not face the world still looking like a patient.

"There's only one thing to do, Phil," someone said. "Hold your breath." Phil breathed as deeply as he could while we tugged on the zip. Slowly, up it went.

"Now hold it just there when you meet the crowd. We don't want it coming down again."

We were trembling with excitement and so, I was sure, was Phil—inside. But he suppressed his excitement as he didn't want to get too impassioned in the dramatic moment. He himself realised that would be harmful to him.

Outwardly I was bubbling over with the joy of the occasion, but inwardly I wondered how Phil was going to take the whole experience. For two-and-a-half months he had led a secluded life; he had virtually no visitors from the outside world except me and then he had seen only my eyes.

Like everybody's big baby, they dressed him up in his blazer and put him in the wheelchair. I thought seldom was such a fuss made of a patient. He wanted to walk, but they said: "No, no, conserve your energy."

Down the passage we went, to the elevator. As we rode down, hasty preparations were made for the meeting with the crowd.

"Don't let anybody see the wheelchair. Once we get within sight of the door, whip away the wheelchair."

I couldn't take my eyes off him, dressed in trousers and a blazer and no longer just pajamas. He looked like a real man again. A well man. A whole man. My man. Off to the door he walked, firmly on his feet. He was ready to meet the crowd.

I shall never forget the dignity with which he faced that audience. He was not nervous. He was not jittery. He was in complete control of himself. He sniffed. "Fresh air, glorious fresh air." What a man, the newspapers wrote, what a man, what a man!

As he stood there self-possessed, self-confident, I wept quietly at the superb mastery he had shown in the situation. It must have been an ordeal for him. For he was not Philip Blaiberg the actor, he was Philip Blaiberg the quiet, hard-working dentist, the man who shunned crowds at parties,

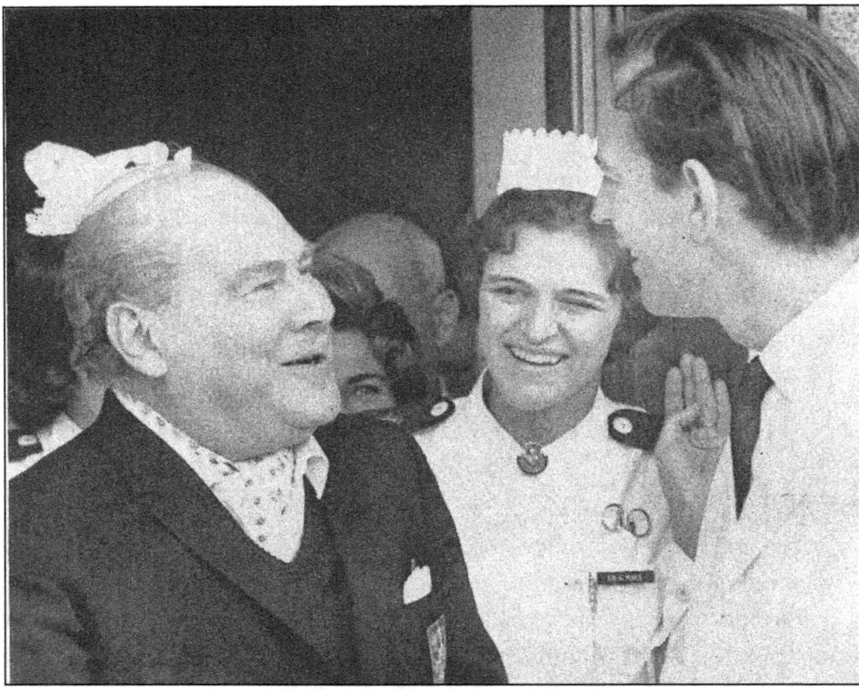

Phil says goodbye to Barnard as he leaves the hospital.

who preferred to read a good book than attend a cocktail party.

From that moment right to the end he seemed to be able to take in his stride the adulation heaped on him. Maybe I am prejudiced, but I like to think he became the darling of the world for the natural, uncomplicated, unaffected way in which he accepted the adulation of the people.

He never changed as a result of the operation. He was the same Philip Blaiberg. It was this aspect that appealed so much to everybody.

"How fantastic that you could keep your head when all about you were losing theirs," someone wrote about Phil's appearance on television.

As we got into the car that day and the crowd pushed around us on every side and the photographers climbed over one another to get their pictures I thought that this happiness could not last. One day, and it would be all gone. But it lasted for another 17 months.

A police escort led us all the way to our apartment in Wynberg. Along the way people lined the streets and they waved and they cheered as we passed them. So this is what it feels like to be royalty. I was in a dream

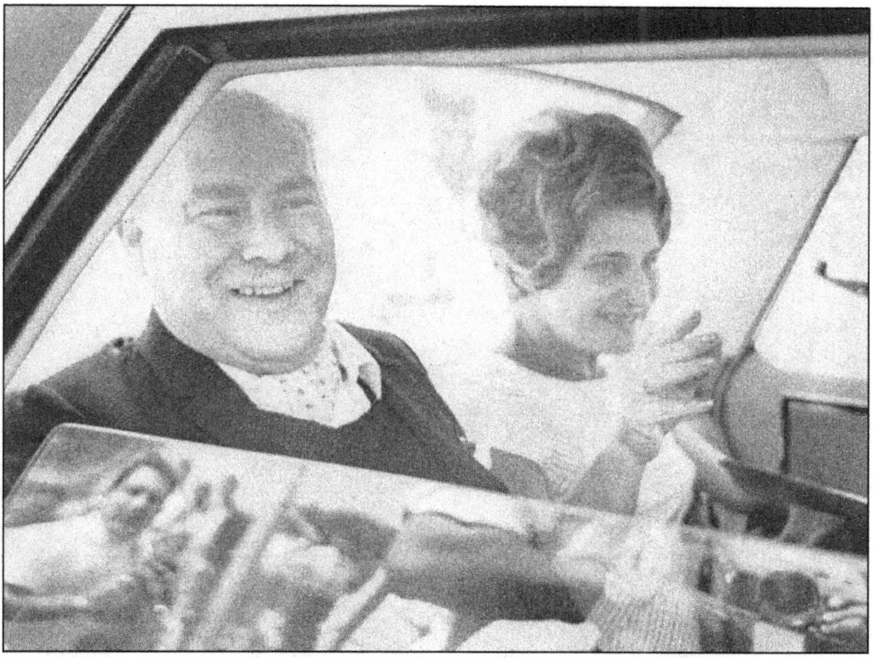

Car mobbed on way home

world. Phil, too, was in a dream world—but a different one from mine.

"Isn't it all so beautiful—the trees, the mountains, the fresh air," he said. "I just can't believe that once more I am going home."

We shared one feeling. That was gratitude.

Gratitude for those who had made this possible, the doctors, the nursing staff, the hospital authorities.

Gratitude for the policemen who would be posted at our door for a week, ensuring us peace and quiet as we were lost in the joy of sharing life again together.

Gratitude, too, for our domestic servant Katie, waiting faithfully in the apartment for us.

Phil looked around him. "Gee, it's a wonderful world. What a wonderful world to be in. What a wonderful home to be back in."

What happened after that is history. Our every movement was reported in the newspapers as an astonished and fascinated world tried to recover from their shock of discovering that a man was living with someone else's heart stitched into his body.

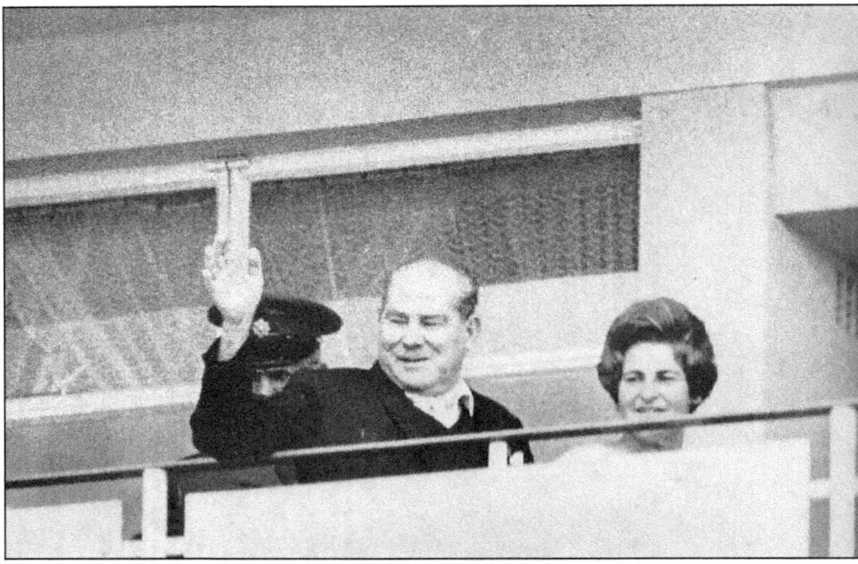

Greeting the crowd from the balcony

As we settled down to a more-or-less normal life, we still had to guard against the danger of infection. For three weeks Phil was allowed no visitors, not even members of our family. For the whole of his post-operative life I was not allowed to kiss Phil. The last kiss we shared was before he underwent the transplant.

The only way Phil could greet our friends and members of our family was to go on to the balcony and wave to them as they stood in the courtyard below. We often joked about this and said he was like the Pope giving an address to his audience. As more and more people gathered around below he would talk and wave to them all.

The first person Phil wanted to see was Dorothy Haupt, widow of the man whose heart was put in Phil's body.

It was an historic moment in our lives when she came to see us. But, for all the drama it might intrinsically have contained, it was little more than an ordinary meeting.

Phil said, "I don't know how I can thank you enough for giving your permission for the transplant so readily so I can be here today."

Mrs. Haupt looked at him with admiration. I wondered what was going through her mind. Was it psychological as she thought whose heart was keeping him alive, or was it just because Phil was Phil? She and Clive's mother thought a great deal of him.

In addition, the doctors said we could have one reporter and one photographer who relayed all our news to the world from the start so that we could keep the crowd happy.

(Graham Fysh, the co-author of this book, was that reporter and Jim McLagan was the photographer. They both worked for The Cape Argus.)

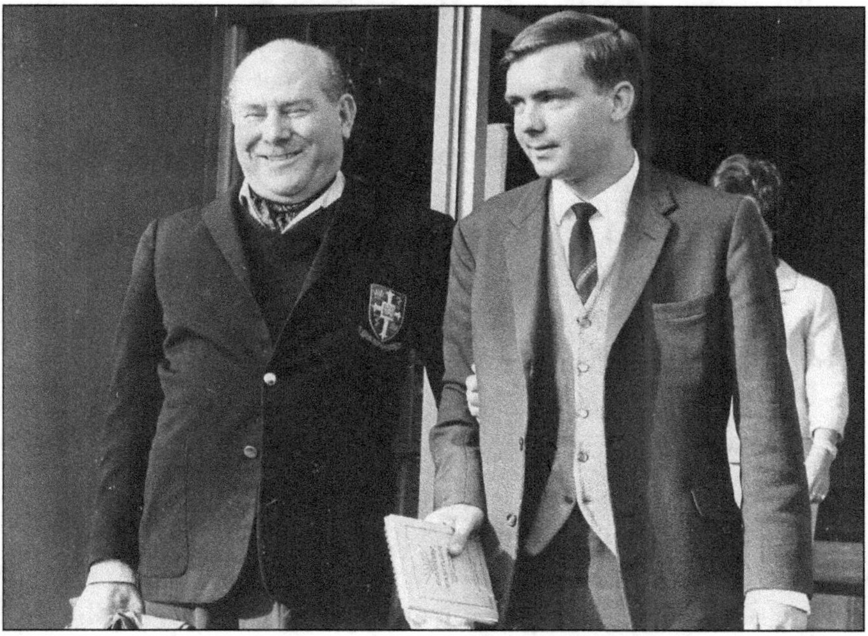

Phil with reporter Graham Fysh, notebook in hand. (Photograph by Jim McLagan)

Later my brother and sisters were allowed to see him. Gradually more people were allowed to see us, just a few at a time, until we got to our normal routine—our normal routine after the transplant, that is, for more than six people were not allowed to be with Phil at one time. The doctors warned us to beware of infection.

At the beginning I watched him like a mother hen watching her chickens, but it was rarely necessary.

All the instructions I had from the nurses about the medicines were rather laughable, because, in his methodical, efficient way, Phil took over that duty completely.

At meal times, he would take out a notebook and then write down the pills he had taken at each meal. He took his own temperature three times a day. I learned I should have no fear of having to do any nursing as I had feared. He looked after himself well. But I still kept a watchful eye on him.

"You must stop watching me like this, Eileen. You must remember that I am a healthy, well man." In fact, he became annoyed if anybody thought of him as anything different.

When, after six weeks, he was permitted by the doctors to leave the flat for drives and walks on the mountain and beach, he would inevitably be stopped by someone who would say: "But, Dr. Blaiberg, do you think you should be out now? It is getting a little chilly, you know?" or some such remark, occasioned undoubtedly by genuine concern for Phil's well-being.

His reactions to these remarks were the first times I saw him losing his temper. All our lives he had been patient, but remarks that implied he was not normal would infuriate him.

"Look," he would say. "I have a team of the best doctors in the world looking after me, will you all stop giving me advice?"

His anger became so serious to us that one evening my brother and I sat down with him and explained to him that that was human nature.

People thought of him as something fragile. All right, they were wrong, but could he not accept that they were thinking only of his good? He promised to try to get used to the idea.

I tried to reason with him on another point. "To you, Phil, the heart is just a pump, to you it was a normal thing, although it was an outstanding medical achievement. But the layman cannot get used to the idea of a man with a new heart. It is the seat of all emotions as far as people in general are concerned. They can't accept a heart transplant as something run-of-the-mill. They can't help it. To them you are different —you'll just have to accept the concern they show for you and the advice they give you."

Grudgingly he learned to live with this.

I joked later with Phil that he was becoming something of a spoiled boy. When he walked down the street, everyone would recognise him and stop to speak to him or greet him.

Phil was not at home long when we realised you could not stop the admiration of the world at what had happened to him.

Presents poured in from all parts of the world. Our mail flood increased to emergency proportions. Local people gave us gifts.

15

Earlier, Phil was determined to mount a major hurdle before leaving hospital. He was determined to walk properly before he returned home to face the world again. But it was something he would never be able to do.

The doctors felt they could not say to him: "You are never going to walk again the same way as you did before." They were hoping he would realise this himself.

One day a doctor said to him: "Dr. Blaiberg, I think you are ready to go home." "Oh no you don't," he said. "I will not go home until I am walking properly."

"You know, Dr. Blaiberg, it might take a long, long time."

"I am not facing the world as a cripple."

It was quite a problem.

Professor Barnard reasoned with Phil. "Try a walking stick. I know you are a proud old devil, but there's nothing wrong with it. You will start off with it and gradually it will be dropped and you will see how much you will improve."

It took a few days' persuasion before Phil said: "All right. I will go home with a stick."

Afterwards I realised how much of this was not just plain pride in himself, but it was pride in Professor Barnard, the heart team and Groote Schuur, which became all-important to him.

He was their advertisement. People should not be able to say he was not 100 percent well.

After he had returned home, he would make a joke of the cane.

When photographers wanted to take pictures of him, he would say: "Eileen, take away the walking stick, I don't want them to see it."

Hiding it behind his back, he would add: "We are not going to let Chris Barnard down. I want to give a decent showing to the world. I am a well man. They must not know about the stick."

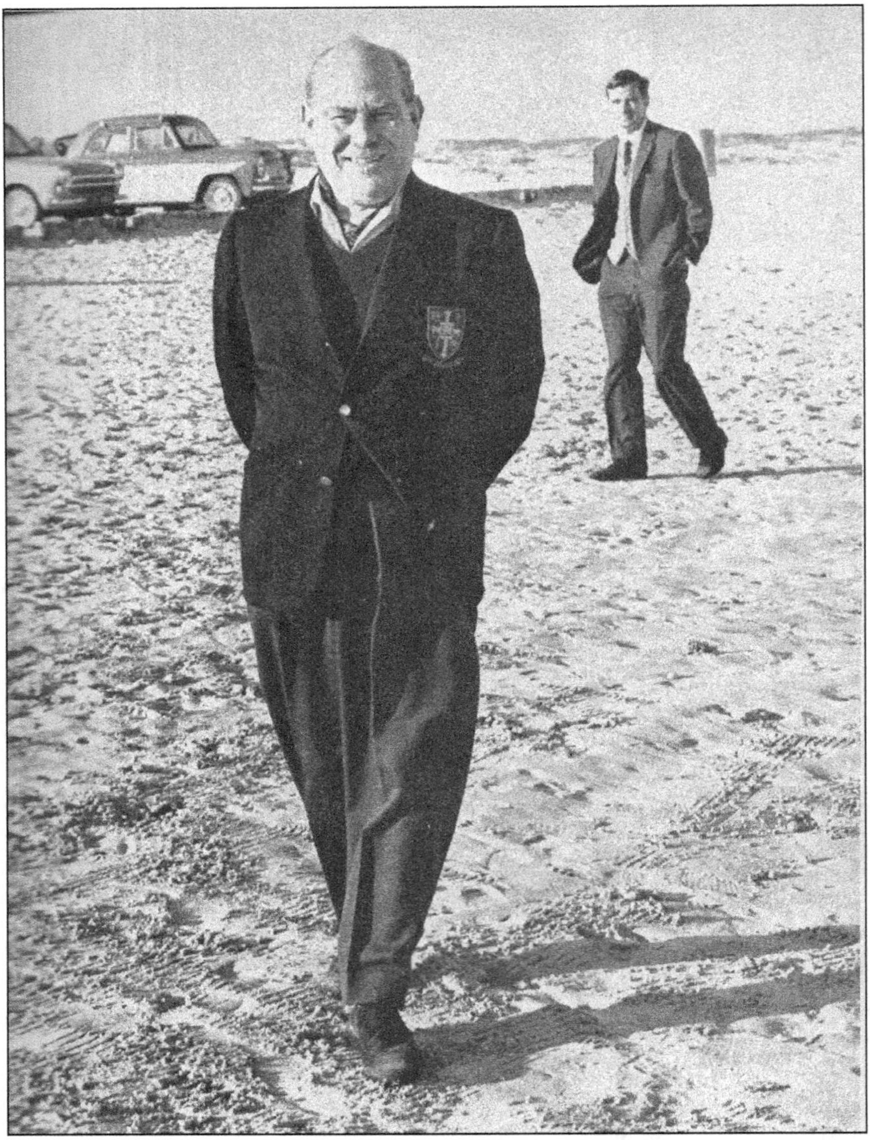

Phil walks on Muizenberg beach. (Graham Fysh in background.)

Although he could walk a short distance without the stick, he never really got rid of it. He always needed it from that day he left the hospital to the time he died. His legs never really got right again. It is to his credit that the world never found out how bad his legs really were.

Actually, we thought it was his legs, but afterwards I learnt that it was his back that was the cause of the trouble.

I heard almost every day: "Isn't it fantastic, can you see how much better I am walking?"

It was an illusion on his part. His walking never improved. In his mind it did. That was what really mattered. It made him happy and it gave him a goal to which he could strive.

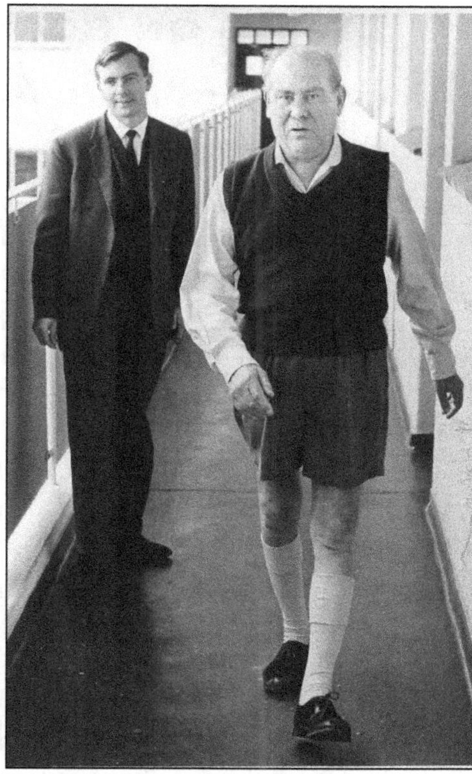

Phil in the passage alongside his apartment showing he can walk without a stick.

Because it made him happy, it made me happy, too.

For 11 months he said: "You will see next week I'll be climbing those steps alone."

Always it was going to be next week. But for 44 weeks next week never came.

Intelligent a man as he was, he never realised that he was not improving—unless I am the fool and he was trying to bluff me.

Although I knew he was not as well again as he was when he was home for the first time after the transplant, all that mattered was that he was so happy.

He was determined to fight all the time without complaining.

To illustrate his general state of mind, here's a copy of a column that appeared in newspapers around the world on April 10, 1968 as part of the *Dr. Blaiberg Day by Day* series.

LIVING ON BORROWED TIME

Day by day, Dr. Blaiberg is doing more and more

By Dr. Philip Blaiberg

FRIENDS WHO HAVE known me well have often said to me: "Phil, Why can't you be more optimistic? Why do you always expect the worst?" Today you'd be surprised just how optimistic I feel.

A week ago I did expect the worst, I admit that during the first few days at home I approached life in a fatalistic way. As I explained then, I pondered how long all this exhilarating progress in my physical condition would last.

But it has lasted. More important, the functioning of my organs—my kidneys, my lungs, liver and new heart become more efficient every day. I have not yet suffered a setback.

Nothing appears to have gone wrong. Quite the contrary. Each day I conquer new goals which once I thought to be several weeks distant.I can now lower myself into a squatting position, when I want to tie my shoelace for example, and get back up again with relative ease. Four days ago this would have been impossible.

(But Eileen did get a slight scare the other morning when I toppled over just as I was desperately trying to raise myself into a standing position.)

You may well ask what sort of achievement this is. Why should I feel some pride in being able to lift a heavy jug of water with one hand?

Please try to remember that I started to use the relevant muscles in my arms and legs only a few weeks ago.Prior to that these muscle tissues had lain dormant and had started to waste away during the many months of my illness. I hate repeating myself, but it was last November that I was desperately ill and ultimately bedridden for almost three months.

When that happens all the powerful muscles you may once have had slowly degenerate.

So if I start boasting about physical movements that you perform hourly without thinking, forgive me. But the pleasure I get out of seeing my arms and legs return to their normal function is boundless.

Spare time for me a second, and drop this newspaper on the floor. Then pick it up again. While that effort may have been a waste of your time, to me it is a valuable exercise in rehabilitation. For when I do it I have to concentrate hard and control my movements, and in doing so I can feel my neglected muscles twitching back into life.

Many people have written to me asking for more clinical detail on my progress. Their requests are fully justified, I suppose, provided they are prompted by genuine interest and not simply morbid curiosity.

I will try to answer some of them as best I can. What I cannot, and will not, answer are some of the thoroughly ludicrous queries I receive. For example, I received a query the other day from someone who asked if I thought any differently or experienced any unusual and foreign emotions following the implantation of a new heart inside my chest.

That letter, I'm afraid, was promptly filed in the wastepaper basket. Surely any rational being must recognize that the medieval belief that the heart is the seat of the soul is now no more than the romantic fancy of the poets.

Any clinical description of my present situation must be brief, for there is very little to tell. Every day I take my variety of medicines, ranging from the antacids and vitamins to the immunosuppressive drugs and digitalis—those long established drugs and digitalis serve to stimulate the muscles of my new heart.

Last week I told you I was taking 18 pills a day. I was wrong. A quick recount shows the grand total to be 30. I do not suffer any annoyance from them at all. What I do suffer is the rather unpleasant taste that these drugs can often leave in the saliva. Whether it is the immunosuppressive pills, the Immuran or the Prednisone, I don't know.

This is a very trivial discomfort, however, that I gladly tolerate. As for the new heart, it has a firm and steady beat and does everything that I require of it.

Today I have had the privilege of coming to terms with life. I labour under no false illusions. I realise that there are vast stretches of the unknown that I have yet to explore. My feelings are best expressed by those immortal lines of Shakespeare: "To thine own self be true, And it must follow, as the night the day, Thou canst not then be false to any man."

Phil had a special visitor on April 28, 1968. The world-famous American pianist Liberace, touring South Africa, toasted Phil and told him that he, too, had experienced a near-death experience. Priests administered last rites for him in 1963 when he suffered acute kidney failure through inhaling toxic fumes, he told Phil, but he responded well to the treatment he was given.

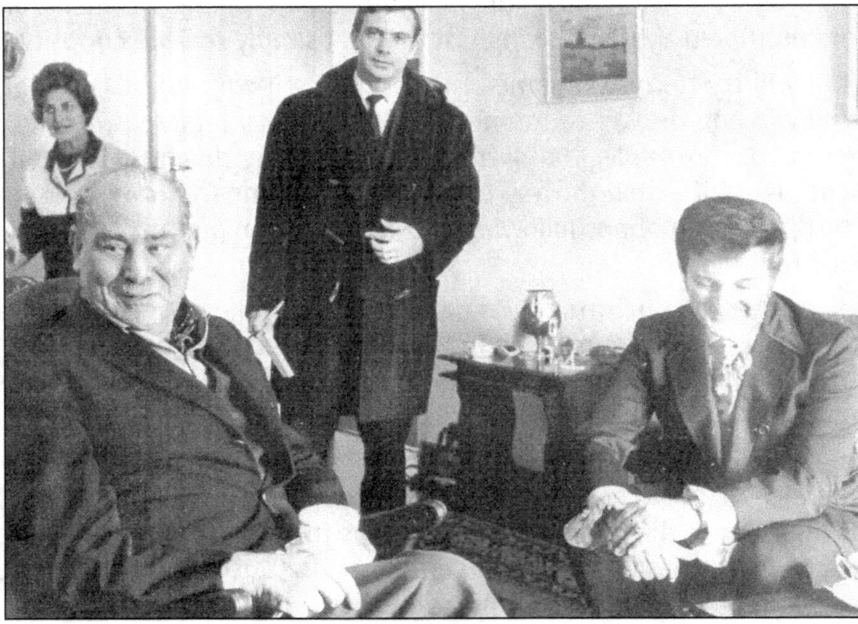

Eileen, Phil, reporter Graham Fysh, and Liberace in the Blaiberg home.

You had to live with Phil during this time to understand the courage he had. Let me tell you this story as an example.

One bright summer's day we went to a beach on the Atlantic ocean where Phil wanted to swim. The tide was high, sweeping in over the rocks. In order to get to the water, Phil had to walk some distance with his stick—but he was shy to do this alone. No one should know that he could not walk unaided. So he asked me to walk with him and to pretend that we were holding hands simply out of affection for each other. He took the walking stick too, hut acted as though it was not important.

I thought that Phil would ask me to walk with him to the sheltered tidal pool where he could have a quick dip in the water and then return. Imagine my surprise when he led me towards the open sea and the breakers bounding in between the rocks.

He did not stop at the edge of the water either. He went in deeper and deeper, in spite of my protests. I had to accompany him as I did not want him to be stranded without any help.

When I look back now I can see the humorous side to that incident. There was Phil, walking deeper and deeper into the sea, clutching his walking stick in one hand and me in the other hand.

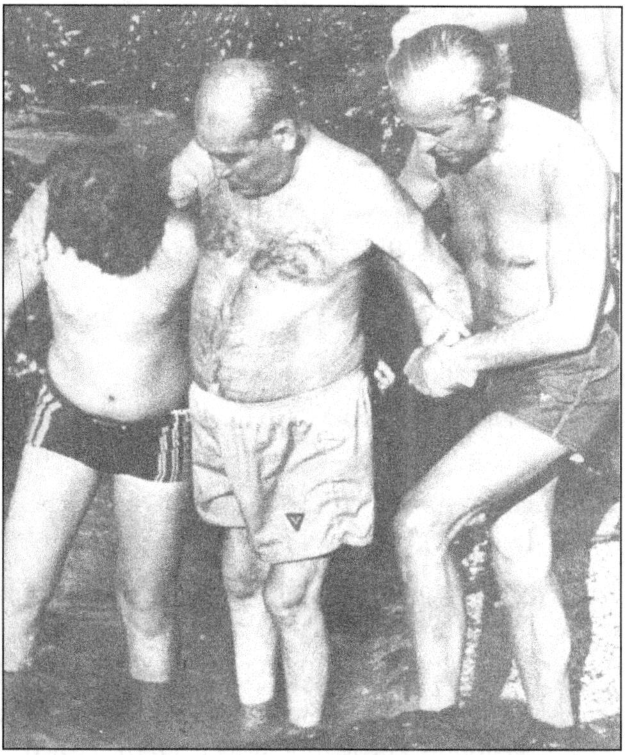

Phil is helped out of the water.

Everybody on the beach was watching him for, of course, they had recognised him even before he went into the water.

Youngsters, particularly, were fascinated. Fortunately some people noticed how Phil was dragging me in farther and farther. They must have seen the look of fear on my face for they told me afterwards that they sensed I was nervous.

Two men came into the water to help both of us to come out again. Phil became annoyed with them, saying he did not need any help.

I quickly said that I was the one who needed help and that the men had come to help me. Besides anything else, the water was cold, the beach being on the Atlantic side of the Peninsula, where the water is generally noticeably colder than that on the Indian Ocean side.

Phil handed the man his stick, then to everybody's amazement he dived under the water. Then he got up out of the water and the man helped him out. There was a big grin on Phil's face as he reached the shore.

I could imagine him saying, "I'll show them what Philip Blaiberg is made of. I'll show them I'm as normal as anyone else."

But he would not do anything for exhibitionism. He would do it only if he wanted to do so.

Suddenly it struck me that day that it would be impossible for us to swim on a beach like that. It was a scene that was likely to be repeated every time Phil visited the beach—people swarming about us asking for Phil's autograph.

Next time we tried the Sea Point Pavilion which consists of open-air swimming baths. Phil said he would like that because he would be able to swim properly there.

But there the crowds were even worse. Even more children crowded round him asking for his autograph.

Then we made a vow that the Atlantic side of the coast would have to be taboo for us because there were too many people there.

I became angry with the people because they would not leave Phil alone, but Phil kept encouraging them.

When we got home I told Phil that he was not getting any relaxation. At home his time was taken up writing letters and at the beach it was taken up with the signing of autographs. He agreed that he was a little tired.

After these incidents we went to the Indian Ocean side of the coast where we found a little spot away from the crowd.

Although people came to speak to Phil when we sat there, they were more disciplined, mainly because they consisted of adults, whereas there were far more children on the beaches on the Atlantic side.

Occasionally I would hint to people that Phil was feeling tired and they would soon leave. There was not that jostling that we experienced on the Atlantic coast.

The spot that we chose afterwards became known as "Blaiberg Corner."

People would often walk past just to look at Phil.

The next event I remember with particular happiness was his re-birthday—one year after he underwent the transplant. He looked so well at the time even though he was still walking with a stick.

The preparations for his re-birthday made December 1968 a particularly busy month.

Reporters and television newsmen came from all parts of the world to interview him in readiness to release the interviews on that day. He was busy from morning to night being interviewed. He did it willingly and gladly.

One of the films taken at that time was given to Phil as a gift afterwards. It was a wonderful record of his post-operative life.

In that film, believe it or not, he never appeared once with that walking stick. The crew took two weeks to film it.

On some occasions they took him out alone, without me to hold his hand and so give him some support. But he always appeared without the stick.

I must admit that at times he was a bit wobbly on his feet, but nothing more than that.

That effort became a great tribute to him. I recall particularly the joy with which he spoke. He was loving life so much.

In fact, we had many letters from America as a result of the interview in that film.

Indeed, many tributes that we received after he died came in as a result of that film. He made a great impression in it.

Once more it was because he was himself. When he answered questions he never tried to impress anybody. He did not rehearse anything either; it was simply a film taken of him as he was.

What summed up his whole character, to my mind, in that film was when the newsman asked him: "Do you feel any different?"

He treated the whole thing lightly, saying "No, the heart is just a pump."

On that day—January 2, 1969—we went to the beach as usual. When we walked on to it, everybody in the vicinity started clapping, remembering that it was Phil's re-birthday. They came up and said how happy and proud they were for Phil.

When it came to lunchtime crowds gathered around us. I appealed to them: "Please let him have his re-birthday lunch in peace."

They all said I was quite right to make that request and they went off within a few minutes without there being any trouble at all.

Jill, Phil and I were all due to go overseas in March or April, 1969. Phil was terribly excited. Optimist that he was, he planned to try to fit all he wanted to see into four weeks.

"That is more than a healthy man could do," the travel agent told Phil.

I squirmed. I knew how Phil felt about statements like that.

"I am healthier than most men," Phil replied.

I tried to rescue the situation. "Perhaps you can manage it darling, but I will not be able to do all that in four weeks."

"Well, I will drag you along then."

Later the tour was lengthened to six weeks. Fortunately the travel arrangements had to be vetoed by Professor Barnard. When the agent sent him the plan, Professor Barnard just laughed. He said Phil would have to shorten it from six weeks to a month because it was too long.

At first Phil said, "I am my own boss, I will decide where I want to go." But that didn't last for long because he quickly realised that he owed it to the transplant team to listen to them in case anything went wrong on the trip.

As the time for us to go on the trip drew nearer, I could see that the doctors were getting more and more worried about it. They didn't say very much, but I could see they were not enthusiastic.

A doctor said he would be happier if Phil didn't go, but Phil said it was a lot of nonsense, he would take his own doctor with him. It was left to "Bossie" (Dr. Bosman) to rectify the situation.

"I am not going to sleep for a whole month while you are away," he told Phil. "I have encouraged you up to now, "but if you want to do me a great favour, don't go."

"If that is the way you feel, Bossie, I am not going."

Bossie himself was taken aback with Phil's quick reply.

He could not get over his quick submission. He had not realised up to then how much sway he had over Phil and how much Phil relied on his judgment. I think it was because Bossie never ordered Phil, but told him things in a pleasant, tactful sort of way.

I could not hide my disappointment when I heard the trip was off because I had never been overseas.

I was looking forward so much to the trip. But I soon brushed my disappointment aside. Phil's health came first. Maybe he would be able to go one day.

But the next day Phil said he was determined that I should go overseas.

"I will never leave you," I told him.

"Well if you don't go I will divorce you."

I felt I needed that break badly. But I would never have gone had he not forced me to do so.

I telephoned my sister in Port Elizabeth, asked her to come with me and she agreed. We decided to leave on March 31.

We went away for a month. I didn't have to write one letter in preparation for the trip, nor did I have to arrange anything. Phil saw to it all. And he had fun doing it, too.

I felt sad about it because had Phil gone the trip would have been funded by television and other companies abroad.

Now that he was not going, however, we had to pay for it ourselves. I told Phil that I was causing him a lot of extra expense.

"No, you go and enjoy yourselves. Ever since we were married I have dreamed of the day you would go overseas.

"I always hoped I would be there to see your face, but I want to be alive still while you go overseas so I get pleasure at knowing you have been."

I maintained contact with Phil while I was overseas by telephoning him twice a week. I was able to do this through the co-operation of newspapers whose reporters interviewed me.

Whenever I telephoned, he said he had never been so well. It was almost as though he was better without me.

When I returned, however, I realised that he had said this so that I would enjoy my holiday more.

When I returned I saw for the first time the retrogression that had taken place in him. I was taken aback when I saw him.

I had been away for four weeks, but I could notice the difference in him. It was like a child growing up—his mother does not notice how much he is growing, but someone who sees him only occasionally does.

Now I saw Phil with objective eyes. And I was shocked.

"You look well," I said, trying to look enthusiastic.

But from that day to the day he died, I was never happy, about Phil's condition. A gradual retrogression was taking place from which he would never recover.

16

It was about a month before Phil died that Professor Chris Barnard posed the most difficult question I have ever been asked to answer.

"Your husband is very ill," he said to me.

"We really don't want him to die, he is somebody so special in our lives. Will you consider giving permission for him to have another transplant?"

I replied that I was not eager, but when the time came we would see what Phil thought. I was not in favour of it because I felt that he had suffered enough.

About a week later, when Phil was in a jocular mood, I said to him: "If they wanted to perform another transplant on you, what would you feel about it?"

"What's the difference?" he said. "If ole Chris wants it to make him happy, let him have it."

He spoke as though he was the most irrelevant person in the whole affair.

Then three weeks later, just seven days before Phil died, Professor Barnard put the question to me again.

"It is now or never," he said. "I know you are not keen, but it is his only chance."

I thought of what Phil had said. But I thought, too, of the excruciating stomach pain that Phil had been suffering recently. He had never had pain like that previously. It was almost unbearable to watch him suffer.

I thought of Phil struggling to live and I answered.

"The answer is emphatically no."

After I said that, however, my conscience began worrying me. Maybe I had taken away his only chance of living and I had taken away my only chance of having my husband with me.

Who could help me in my dilemma?

Who was there who knew and understood the problem? Who was there who knew Phil as well as I did and could look at it from the point of view of what was best for him?

I turned for advice to Katie, our domestic servant.

"Katie, they want to give him another new heart. What do you think?"

"Madam, please don't say yes. Doctor's had as much as he can take. He has suffered enough, just take it this time and let him rest peacefully."

My conscience troubled me no longer. My dilemma had been solved.

I went back to Professor Barnard.

"You might think it is funny that I should take advice from my domestic servant, but she loves him as much as I do. And she says no."

The doctors never asked me that question again.

When all this happened we had already moved into our new house in Newlands. Phil was happy here. He loved this house in which Jill and I still stay.

Because he loved it, I love it, too.

Phil tried hard to get his papers in order and to write. But as hard as he tried it was a tremendous battle to get anything done.

After sitting at his desk for five hours he would say that he had written three letters. In happier days he had finished 30 to 40 in that time.

But, amazingly enough, these stark facts that illustrated so tellingly his failing health never penetrated to him. He kept thinking he was getting better.

During those last few weeks Phil was more emotional than I had ever known him to be before.

He would cry easily, something he would never have done in his pre-transplant life and even in those earlier days after the operation. He had always been tough, as hard as concrete in the face of upset.

Phil's deterioration became noticeably worse about 10 days before he died.

A night nurse came to attend to him. She would turn him and tend to him during the night.

I told her that if Phil had a bad turn she should call me immediately.

At this stage he had to sleep in a room on his own. He did not want to be in the room with me in case he disturbed me, he said. And I thought he would be more comfortable on his own.

On Sunday, August 10, I went to bed as usual after saying goodnight to him. Early on the following morning the nurse aide came into my room.

"Telephone the oxygen people quickly. His supply of oxygen is running out." Since May we had a cylinder of oxygen in the house in case Phil should require it in an emergency.

"It is nearly empty?"

"Yes he has been using oxygen since 2 a.m."

"Since 2 a.m.? But you promised to call me should he need assistance."

"Every time I tried to come to your room, doctor would say: 'Don't wake Mrs. Blaiberg. She will need all the rest she can get because I am in for a bad spell'."

Can you imagine any other person thinking like that? I would think that most people in a situation like that would panic and call their nearest relative immediately. But Phil was made of stronger stuff than that. His first thought was that I should have rest.

As I thought of what he had done, of the concern he had shown for me when he was scarcely able to breathe, my anger dissipated and in its place was a big lump in my throat—a lump of admiration and love.

I could hardly speak on the telephone to ask for the extra oxygen. The lump made it difficult.

After telephoning, I ran in to his room to see how he was. He put up a brave face once more. But I was terribly distressed when I saw him.

I knew it was near the end.

I turned then to the man who had meant so much to both of us and was to mean so much in the next few days—Bossie.

"Phil has been on oxygen all night, what do I do?"

"Nothing. I will be there in a few minutes."

Fifteen minutes later Bossie was there. And he lives a half-an-hour's drive away from our house.

I knew how I could get a good objective indication of Phil's condition. It was by looking at Bossie's face when he saw him. I looked, read the message—and I knew things were bad. Bossie could not hide what he felt because by then Phil had become more like a brother to him than a patient.

He telephoned Professor Barnard, Dr. Marius Barnard, Chris's brother, and Dr. Alan Conlan, who had been looking after Phil at various times.

From 8 o'clock that morning the others started arriving. On each face I read the same message of distress.

We sat on the patio at the back of the house and discussed what was best.

They told me then that Phil's days were numbered. Could this really be the end? It seemed too impossible to believe. Twice I had thought there was no hope for him and twice he had proven me a pessimist.

Also, once before the doctors had told me there was no hope for him—and Phil had lived for another year. Perhaps they were being unduly realistic again, perhaps there was still a chance.

And yet something told me there was nothing now that could save Phil. Instinctively I knew this to be true.

Yet I felt there was that chance. He could live, couldn't he? He could pull through again, just as he pulled through before, couldn't he?

Even as I asked myself those questions I knew they were no more than rhetorical.

My thoughts were brought down to earth as Professor Barnard spoke.

"I think the important thing is where he would be happiest—here at home or in the hospital. I don't think he will come out of this alive wherever he is."

"There is no question in my mind," I replied. "If there is a choice, I would like him to stay here, to die here in this house he adores so much."

From the Monday to the Wednesday of that week the house was seldom empty. We had five or six people for lunch every day. He was so ill at that time—so desperately ill—that there was always someone from the hospital in our house.

As he lay there, a dying man, one person kept up our spirits—that person was Phil himself. The nurses could hardly believe their ears when they heard him telling us jokes and keeping us amused.

On Thursday morning, Phil was taken to the hospital. Then, for the first time, the newspapers heard he was so ill.

The ironical part of that was that the reason Phil was taken to hospital was that he was slightly better on the Thursday. His blood count and his pulse rate had both improved.

The doctors felt it was safe to take him to the hospital then—and it was imperative, too, as they could care for him better there.

At a time when the world heard of Phil's illness for the first time and everyone started thinking: "He has taken a sudden turn for the worse," I started thinking: "Perhaps he is on the road to recovery."

Strange things started happening then.The hospital staff told me that clinically Phil was a little better, and yet by Thursday his condition had so that deteriorated—so much he could hardly speak. He seemed worse to me, yet according to the statistics, he was a little better.

The doctors were still worried, but they said he was showing a slight improvement To me the outlook was bleak. But I never gave up hope.

It seems to me that things like this are atypical when it comes to transplanted hearts.

When I visited Phil on Sunday afternoon I needed no statistics or doctors to tell me Phil's condition. I could tell immediately that he was close to death.

I will tell you why. He had never spoken about death ever before. Always he had been optimistic. Nevertheless when I walked into his ward that Sunday afternoon, he looked sadly up at me and said, "Eileen, you know I am dying, I am on my way out."

I was stunned. The sister had to help me out of the room.

Now I knew the truth.

When Phil was in the hospital at that time, Professor Barnard could not visit him as he was suffering from a cold.

On that Sunday afternoon he saw me outside the ward. I was crying, "What's the matter?" he asked, "My husband just told me he is dying."

"But that's a good sign. If he says that it means he is getting better."

You don't know my husband, I thought. When he says that it does not mean he is getting better.

I went back into the room and I suggested that we give Phil supper.

For the last few days he had not wanted to eat at all. But I had found that it was no use asking him if he wanted any food. He was so weak that it was best just to give it to him. When you did that, he opened his mouth and ate.

I mentioned we were going to give him supper and Phil said: "All I would like is some cold consommé."

"Right, I will go home and make some." Just then Jill came into the room.

Then again Phil did something he had rarely done before. He stroked Jill and he said: "My baby, my lovely girl." That was unusual because Phil seldom showed his feelings in that way.

It looked a lot like the end to me.

Jill and I went home to make him the soup. We had just turned on the stove when the telephone rang.

It was Bossie.

"Mrs. Blaiberg, I am so sorry. It is all over."

I responded: "I am very glad."

Had you told me years before that I could say a thing like that about my husband, whom I adored, I would have said you were crazy. But he had suffered so much. I had seen the exhaustion written on his face. I had seen him fight to talk.

When I visited him in those last days, he would open his tired eyes and say, "You poor thing, how boring it must be to sit with a man who can't talk to you."

Then he would fall asleep.

I was glad he was gone...for his sake.

Rest had finally come to him, a rest he so richly deserved.

The date of the day on which Phil died was almost uncanny. Phil died on the same day of the year as my father died.

Israel Harris Abel died on August 17, 1935. Philip Blaiberg died on August 17, 1969. Like father, like husband. History repeated itself.

REFLECTIONS ON PHIL

Phil was more than a dentist. He was a counsellor and, in some ways, almost a psychiatrist.

I think of his humanity and innate kindness towards people, no matter who they were.

He never laughed at people because they were seen by other people as different. He never scoffed at them, or made them have complexes. To him the important thing was that they should feel wanted and needed in a hostile world.

All through his life Phil never worked only for money. He worked for humanity. He had a kindness of the sort I have noticed in few other people. If we went to parties he would be most kind and friendly to all who did not fit in with the rest. While everyone else was talking to the people who "mattered," Phil was in a corner talking to those whom everyone else ignored. And those who felt themselves pushed aside or ignored, in turn, always felt that Phil was someone to whom they could turn.

Even after his operation, when he became something of a V.I.P., Phil did not change. Certainly, he liked it when people recognised him in the street and he felt a degree of pride when they would come up and talk to him. But he did not become vain. That was alien to his nature.

I noticed after the operation that Phil was attracting more and more new acquaintances. But the sort of people who were visiting us were the plumbers, the workmen, the carpenters—the people who do an honest day's work with their hands.

For example, we hired a carpenter and a painter to do work in the flat. When I returned home I found them in the lounge talking and drinking with Phil like old friends.

After Phil died, we received hundreds of letters from Phil's former patients saying how much they felt for him and telling how he had been not only a dentist to them, but a friend.

For example, I received a letter from a woman who had been his patient. I wanted to cry when I read it. "I don't think of him as the heart man," she wrote. "I still think of him as the man who listened to all my little worries."

Another thing about Phil: He was honest to a fault. There was nothing secretive about him. I found this out to my chagrin when he was in practice. While others were already putting up their fees, Phil was always afraid of doing so because he felt he might be overcharging, particularly those who could not afford much. When workmen did odd jobs around our home, Phil would always pay them a little more than they quoted him, whether he could afford it or not.

He and my son taught me another thing. I remember one day when I was a young married woman a man came to the door selling apples. As was the custom—and still is—among most women, I bargained with him. When I beat him down by five cents, my husband and son both shouted at me: "Aren't you ashamed of yourself?"

I wanted to know what I had done wrong.

"What's five cents to you?" asked Phil. "It is not much, but I am sure it means a lot to that man."

From that day to this I have never bargained with a door-to-door salesman. After all, when one thinks of it, we can afford those few extra cents more than they can.

My nickname for Phil was "George Washington." He could not lie. I don't remember in the 33 years that we were married that he ever told a lie.

In his work as a dentist, too, Phil was extremely honest. One is always tempted to do something that is not entirely ethical. And, let's face it, there is scope for this in dentistry. But I believe he went to rest with a clear conscience. He always told the patient the exact truth, I am sure of that.

After the war, men who had been privates came to me and said: "Mrs. Blaiberg your husband was one of the few officers in the Army to whom we could go with our troubles. We not only went to him as a dentist, but as an understanding man. He never treated us as inferior, always as a best friend."

Those who felt themselves pushed aside or ignored always felt that Phil was someone to whom they could turn.

In the 19 months that Phil was alive after the transplant, people so often said to me that what struck them so forcibly was that he was a man whom they could really like. There was that hearty smile, that chubby look, that complete lack of fear or thought for himself.

The most wonderful thing to me was that he never became neurotic. He never took advantage of his operation at all to play up to people. The only time he started complaining was near the end and then I knew he did not have long to live.

To live with a man who had been brought back from the brink of death would, one would expect, be living with somebody abnormal.

People have often said: "What a strain you must have been under."

But any strain was created by me. I worried about him although there was never any need to do so.

He never created a strain in the house because he was such a natural person.

For 19 months there was never a day in which there were fewer than 30 letters in the mail. There was always a reason for people to write to him.

He won the heart of the world not just because he was the longest-living heart transplant recipient, but because he was Philip Blaiberg.

I was the luckiest woman in the world, not only through having lived with the first man to come out of hospital with a new heart, but through living with a man of his calibre for so many years.

What I have gained from him is something for which I can never be thankful enough.

When I married him I was little more than a pretty young girl. Whatever qualities I have today have rubbed off him on to me.

It is not every day that someone has the privilege of living with a man who has such high principles as Phil had.

The most important lesson I learned was the right sense of values. That is what I am trying to pass on to my daughter—to be your own natural self and not to be what you are not.

That is the greatest lesson I learned from Phil.

www.ingramcontent.com/pod-product-compliance
Lightning Source LLC
LaVergne TN
LVHW022005200926
848481LV00007B/2247
* 9 7 9 8 9 8 5 4 8 3 6 7 3 *